THE SIBO DIET PLAN

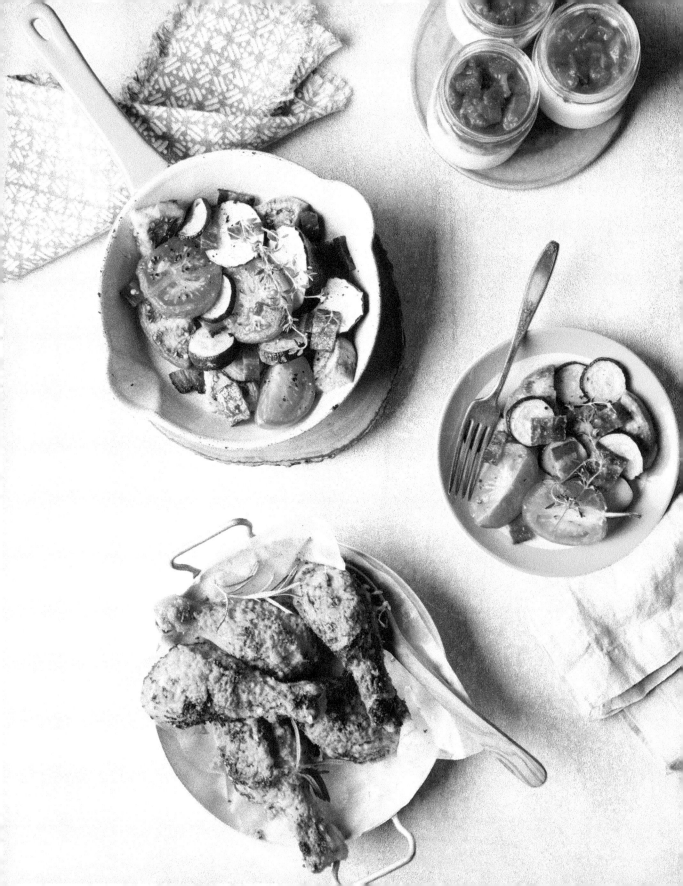

THE
SIBO DIET PLAN

4 WEEKS TO RELIEVE SYMPTOMS AND MANAGE SIBO

Kristy Regan, MScN

Foreword by Allison Siebecker, ND, MSOM, LAc

PHOTOGRAPHY BY MARIJA VIDAL

ROCKRIDGE
PRESS

To my loving and supportive husband, Gregg, and my sweet dog, Zoey—you two make our house a home.

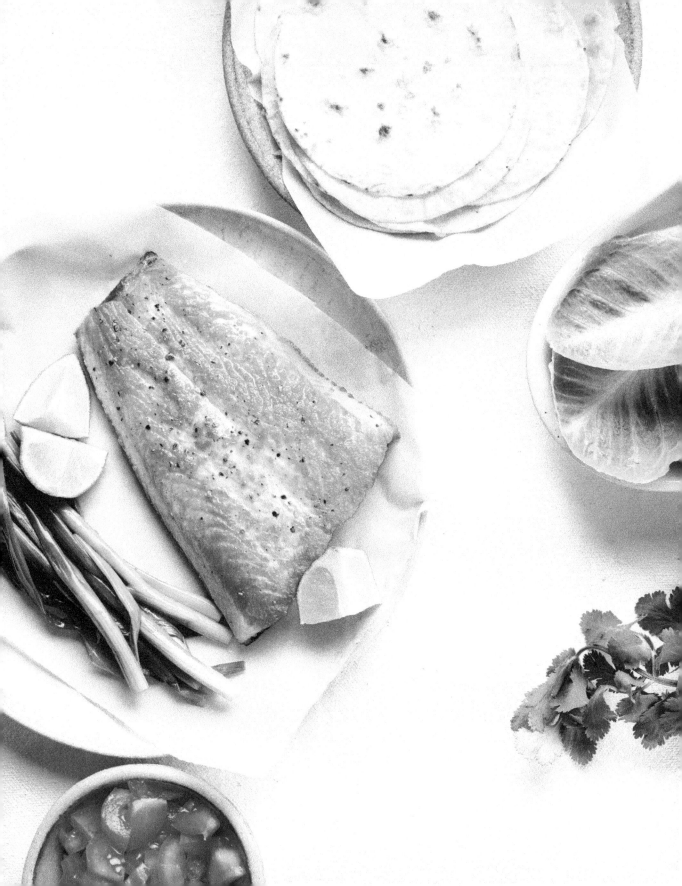

Contents

Foreword

While reading Kristy Regan's *The SIBO Diet Plan*, one quote in particular immediately jumped out: "Avoid adding guilt and fear to your diet." I love that! Eating is an essential part of our social and cultural fabric, and there is no place in food for guilt or fear, no matter what health condition you have. With this book, Kristy offers you a path away from guilt and fear surrounding food and one towards a healthier, happier life with fewer IBS and SIBO symptoms.

I've been living with SIBO since age five. Back then, little did my young self know just how much of a journey SIBO would take me on. As I sought to understand my own condition, I quickly came to realize how many others were affected by SIBO. My personal mission soon became a crusade to help people who, just like me, struggled. Since 2010, I've run a naturopathic practice specializing in SIBO, and I teach advanced gastroenterology focusing on SIBO and IBS at the National University of Natural Medicine in Portland, Oregon, as well as at symposia and conferences all around the world.

In my work, I have taught students, patients, and fellow physicians about SIBO, how it affects IBS, and the role diet plays in its management. For years, I have heard from patients the world over about the negative impact that SIBO and IBS have had on their quality of life. They've also shared their frustration with the restrictive and bland nature of diets that control SIBO, as well as how difficult the diets are to follow and how much intensive prep and cooking is involved. Kristy solves all of these issues in *The SIBO Diet Plan*.

Kristy was one of my students, and I'm proud of what she has to offer in this book. Her approach is simple, practical, and logical, and she makes it as easy as possible for people with busy lives, households, and careers to follow the meal plan, recipes, and tips. Most importantly, the recipes inspire and encourage you to make food enjoyable. Over the years, I've eaten a lot of delicious foods prepared by many of my students and patients following a SIBO diet, and Kristy's food has always tasted the best. I'm delighted she imparts her use of herbs and spices to create mouthwatering flavors.

Books like *The SIBO Diet Plan* can go a long way to help people battling SIBO. As many as 84 percent of patients with IBS have SIBO and, for some, following a SIBO diet eliminates all of their symptoms. One third of people can recover from SIBO completely, while the remaining two thirds may require some type of ongoing dietary

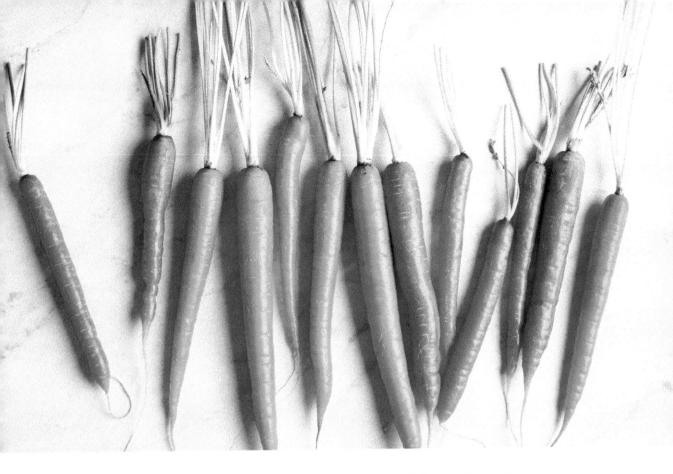

management throughout their lives—however, with dietary changes, their symptoms are vastly improved. Kristy provides options for both types of SIBO patients to find the diet that suits their needs.

I'm also impressed with the simplicity of Kristy's diet plan. The recipes are easy to follow, pantry lists and prep tips are practical time savers, and I appreciate that the meal plan was designed with flexibility in mind, allowing users to personalize their weekly menus according to their dietary and health requirements.

Finally, Kristy has managed to turn a process that is typically stress inducing into a calming solution that is also appetizing and, because of this, *The SIBO Diet Plan* is a new and refreshing source. Even though I've long hosted a SIBO website (SIBOinfo.com) and am in the process of writing my own SIBO book, I find myself really excited to try the plan. And based on my extensive experience treating SIBO patients, this is exactly the kind of positive thinking they need to take charge, stay focused, manage their symptoms, and achieve long-term health and wellness. I know you'll be inspired, too.

—Allison Siebecker, ND, MSOM, LAc

Introduction

LIVING WITH CHRONIC GASTROINTESTINAL SYMPTOMS is, at the very least, challenging, and for many people absolutely life changing. I suffered with IBS symptoms for more than a year before they got extreme enough that I knew I had to address them. I went to see a health practitioner with complaints including diarrhea, flatulence, bowel grumbling, and fatigue. We started with an initial elimination diet that removed gluten and dairy. When those changes didn't mitigate my symptoms, I took a SIBO (small intestinal bacterial overgrowth) breath test. My test came back positive. Upon hearing my diagnosis of SIBO and the prescribed restrictive diet, I was angry, frustrated, and sad. I've always considered myself a gourmand, the person who loves beautiful food, adores cooking, and cherishes communities who come together to share a meal around the table. However, I was determined to take care of my health and well-being, even if it meant changing my life. Over time, I became highly educated about SIBO and, with the help of several instrumental medical practitioners, began to heal. I also made it my mission to help others on their health journeys.

Since there are multiple SIBO diets out there and one isn't universally recognized as the best for everyone, choosing and following a SIBO diet can be confusing and frustrating. I work with clients on many different diets. I see those who have severely limited their diet diversity out of fear, those who are underweight, highly sensitive, and symptomatic—and generally sick and tired. They often follow a severe diet—even when they continue to have unmanageable symptoms—hoping they will eventually feel better. They sometimes lose valuable time going from one diet to another without feeling they've made any progress.

One reason SIBO diets are so confusing is that a diet that is healthy for someone with an intact microbiome will cause symptoms in someone with SIBO. For instance, a high-fiber diet including raw vegetables and whole grains is typically touted as highly beneficial for supporting healthy gut bacteria. But for someone with leaky gut, IBS, or SIBO, it can be difficult to digest hard, raw foods, and high-fiber foods may feed a bacterial overgrowth, causing multiple symptoms. It isn't surprising that people can't figure out the right diet for them, but luckily, there's a better way.

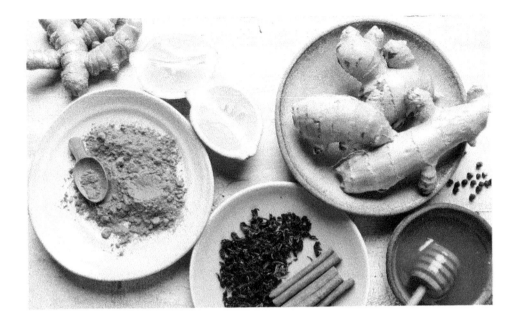

This book outlines a four-week meal plan that includes straightforward and delicious recipes based on a modified low-FODMAP diet. It starts with the most easily digestible foods and builds over the four weeks to include a greater diversity of ingredients prepared in a variety of ways. It simplifies meal planning and preparation, and also offers insights and tips for customizing the diet and troubleshooting suspected food reactions. Since having SIBO can feel isolating, it also addresses choices for eating out with family and friends, socializing at events, and taking a vacation.

My intention in writing this book is to give basic, easy-to-understand information to anyone newly diagnosed with or who suspects they have SIBO. I also provide assistance for those who have been dealing with SIBO for a while but want a fresh perspective and specific dietary information. So, really, this book is for anyone with SIBO or SIBO symptoms. I hope you find something helpful in these pages, whether it's a new recipe, new information, or a new point of view.

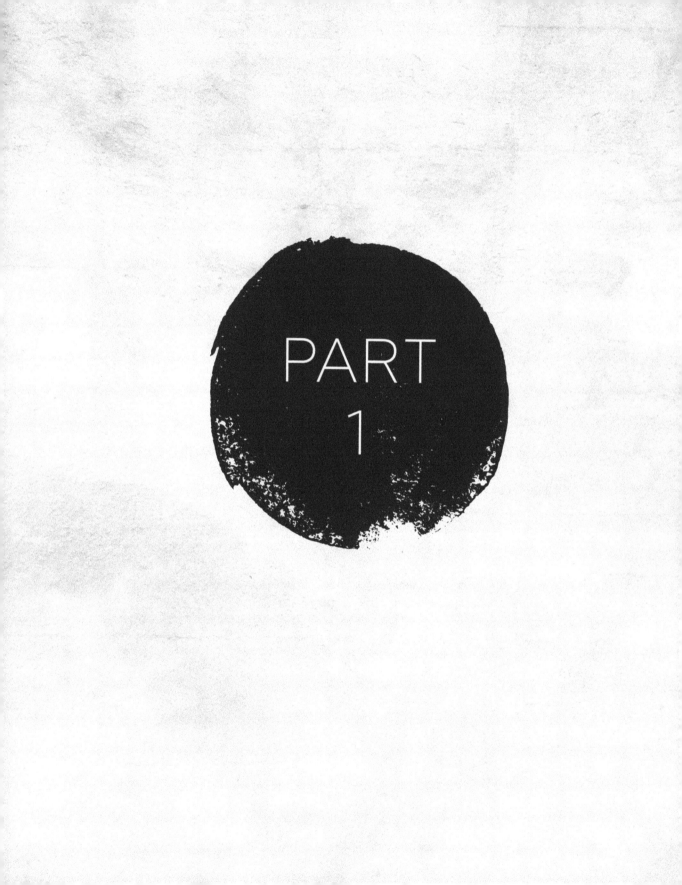

PART
1

Addressing the SIBO Problem

Before embarking on the four-week meal plan, it's important to lay a solid foundation of knowledge regarding what SIBO is, the different types, causes, and symptoms of SIBO, and SIBO testing, diagnosis, and treatment. As many doctors are just becoming aware of SIBO, we also included a quiz to show your doctor, as well as options to consider if you and your doctor don't see eye to eye on SIBO.

SIBO isn't like many other medical issues with only one pharmaceutical choice and one diet. In addition to inconsistent and confusing information, what works for one person may be different for someone else. This book gives consistent and reliable explanations, information, and resources and supports you in becoming an authority on your own health.

After you learn about SIBO, it's time to focus on nutrition and get ready for the four-week meal plan. We will change your home environment and make sure your kitchen is ready with equipment and food items to facilitate a smooth transition. It's important to make sure you're both physically and mentally ready for the transition to a healthy and helpful SIBO diet. Making a commitment to your health in this way leads to increased self-knowledge, a sense of wholeness, and healing.

What Is SIBO?

SIBO stands for small intestinal bacterial overgrowth.

It is an overgrowth of bacteria in the small intestine. Surprisingly, many people, including doctors, have never heard of it. Since symptoms include undesirable gastrointestinal issues such as gas, constipation, or diarrhea, people may feel resistant or ashamed to acknowledge or report their symptoms. If you do talk to your doctor because of increasing symptoms and receding quality of life, you may simply be told to relax or eat more fiber. Alternately, many people are misdiagnosed with IBS. In 2000, Pimentel, Chow, and Lin published their study "Eradication of Small Intestinal Bacterial Overgrowth Reduces Symptoms of Irritable Bowel Syndrome," which showed that in 202 patients with irritable bowel syndrome, 78 percent also had a bacterial overgrowth and, when the overgrowth was cleared, the IBS symptoms disappeared. A 2003 study found that up to 84 percent of people with IBS also have SIBO. Both studies indicate that many people previously diagnosed with IBS actually have SIBO. These findings are spurring additional and much needed research to the underfunded and under-researched areas of IBS and SIBO.

Luckily, many naturopathic doctors (ND) and some medical doctors (MD) have been treating SIBO for many years and continue to refine their treatment. As SIBO begins to be more widely known and research continues on everything from the microbiome to targeted antibiotics to holistic approaches, there is more hope for people who greatly suffer with symptoms every day. This book aims to be part of that support, offering education along with nurturing and delicious recipes that can become household favorites.

THE LOCATION ISSUE

The small intestine is not set up to handle large amounts of bacteria like the large intestine can, so SIBO is, essentially, a location issue. The bacteria aren't necessarily pathogenic, but they are in the wrong place, creating multiple symptoms and nutritional deficiencies.

This bacterial overgrowth in the small intestine can cause damage to the lining of the small intestine, resulting in leaky gut. Once this lining is damaged and becomes permeable, larger proteins move through the lining and cause an immune system reaction, creating food intolerances or allergies. That is why some people get a food intolerance test result that will change over time.

What Causes SIBO?

Normally, there are multiple defenses in place to guard against an overgrowth of bacteria in the small intestine. When one or more of those defenses fails, bacteria aren't cleared from the small intestine, leading to SIBO. A deficiency in the migrating motor complex (MMC) is thought to be the most common cause of SIBO, although altered anatomy, immunodeficiency, ileocecal valve inefficiencies (the ileocecal valve is meant to be a one-way valve, but if it becomes a two-way valve, then waste products from the large intestine can go back to the small intestine), or hydrochloric acid deficiencies can also play a role. The MMC are waves of smooth gastrointestinal muscle contractions that typically perform a cleansing sweep through the small intestine every 90 minutes during periods of fasting. *When the MMC doesn't function properly, bacteria are not cleared in the same manner, setting the stage for an overgrowth.* MMC deficiency is often linked to food poisoning.

Other factors such as stress, use of antibiotics, opiates, or a proton pump inhibitor (PPI), adhesions from prior injuries or surgeries, and chronic diseases like Parkinson's, cancer, hypothyroidism, diabetes, and Ehlers-Danlos syndromes can also play a role. Studies haven't directly linked a poor diet to SIBO, but adopting a diet tailored to limit SIBO symptoms increases quality of life for most people.

Bacteria may also enter the bloodstream, resulting in an immune reaction that can lead to multiple consequences, including chronic fatigue, inflammation, joint pain, headaches, skin rashes such as acne, rosacea, or eczema, brain fog, and memory loss.

In addition to harming the intestinal lining, SIBO causes malabsorption, leading to a variety of deficiencies, including of iron and vitamin B_{12}, resulting in low ferritin or anemia. The bacterial overgrowth may also create bile deconjugation, leading to fatty stools (steatorrhea) and deficiencies in the fat-soluble vitamins, A, D, E, and K. Unabsorbed carbohydrates may draw in water, creating an osmotic effect that can trigger diarrhea. Additionally, the bacteria specifically feed on fermentable carbohydrates and then expel gas, causing a variety of SIBO symptoms including flatulence, belching, GERD, nausea, and bloating. Since the bacteria in SIBO consume carbohydrates, SIBO diets restrict fermentable carbohydrates, and this often results in a dramatic decrease in symptoms.

TYPES OF SIBO

There are several types of SIBO discussed in this section. In the case of hydrogen, methane, or combination SIBO, they won't necessarily affect a person's individual diet but more so will dictate the treatment used for eradicating the SIBO. In the case of hydrogen sulfide SIBO, symptoms may lessen by adopting both a low-FODMAP and a low-sulfur diet. See the Resources (page 206) for a list of high- and low-sulfur foods. This list should be used as a reference only, and individual tolerances should still be tested.

HYDROGEN SIBO

Hydrogen SIBO is connected to an overgrowth of hydrogen gas-producing bacteria. The symptom picture for hydrogen SIBO often includes diarrhea.

METHANE SIBO

It was originally thought that bacteria caused both hydrogen and methane SIBO. But methane gas is produced by Archaea, a single-cell organism lacking a nucleus. Methane-dominant SIBO is connected to symptoms such as constipation, bloating, and flatulence.

COMBINATION SIBO

It is common for people to have a combination of hydrogen and methane SIBO. They may have one type that is more prevalent, or they may have alternating symptoms linked to both hydrogen and methane SIBO.

HYDROGEN SULFIDE SIBO

There currently isn't a SIBO breath test that specifically looks for hydrogen sulfide. Doctors may diagnose hydrogen sulfide SIBO from symptoms and a flat-line breath test. A flat-line breath test often shows numbers for both hydrogen and methane being low (0–2) across the entire test, thus displaying a flat line on the test graph. Symptoms often include sulfur-smelling flatulence, constipation, visceral hypersensitivity, bladder irritation, and an increase in overall SIBO symptoms in conjunction with a high-sulfur diet. If symptoms are not fully indicative of hydrogen sulfide SIBO, it may be helpful to try a low-FODMAP or low-sulfur diet to see whether symptoms recede.

THE TOP COMMON SYMPTOMS

There are numerous SIBO symptoms, including cramping, heartburn, nausea, headaches, memory loss, fatigue, anemia, brain fog, joint pain, and eczema and other skin conditions. Because these can vary and, alone and in combination, negatively affect everyday quality of life, it's important to pay attention to and be aware of your individual symptoms. This makes you an expert on *your health* and better able to work with your health care provider to resolve the issue. Read on for more about the most common symptoms.

CONSTIPATION

Constipation is often linked to a SIBO test that is positive for methane gas. Constipation types vary greatly, but most often people experience decreased bowel movements with a harder consistency. Some people experience constipation followed by a bout of diarrhea, followed by more constipation.

Quiz for the Undiagnosed: Is It SIBO?

1. Do you have any chronic IBS symptoms including diarrhea, constipation, bloating, or abdominal pain?

2. Did your symptoms start or worsen after one or more episodes of food poisoning or stomach flu incidents?

3. Do you have to use medications or supplements such as high-dose magnesium, high-dose vitamin C, or laxatives to have regular bowel movements?

4. Did your symptoms start or increase after surgery?

5. Does your background include frequent antibiotic, opiate, or proton pump inhibitor (PPI) use?

6. Have you adopted a restricted diet to limit symptoms?

7. Do you have anemia or ongoing low ferritin that cannot be attributed to other causes?

8. Does a diet including high-fiber or high-FODMAP foods increase your symptoms?

9. Has a gluten-free diet made little or no discernible difference in your symptoms?

10. Have you noticed improvement in your symptoms when taking antibiotics for a different reason?

11. Have you experienced unwanted weight loss even though you eat the same amount or more?

12. Do you now react to foods you used to be able to eat without any discernible symptoms?

If you answered yes to one or more of these questions, you should make an appointment with your health care provider to be tested for SIBO. Bring this quiz to help start the discussion.

DIARRHEA

Diarrhea as a symptom is often correlated with a positive hydrogen SIBO breath test. Diarrhea varies greatly as well, with some people having many instances of it each day and others having sporadic episodes.

FLATULENCE, BELCHING, AND BLOATING

The gases from a bacterial overgrowth typically cause flatulence, bloating, or belching. When the gases are able to leave your system, they show up either as belching or flatulence. If they are trapped, bloating occurs. This often translates into abdominal distention (looking pregnant by the end of the day) or an uncomfortable feeling of fullness.

FOOD SENSITIVITIES

An intestinal overgrowth of bacteria may cause damage to the small intestine's lining. Thereafter, larger proteins may move through the lining, not fully digested, causing an immune reaction resulting in food sensitivities and other issues.

ANXIETY

Many people with SIBO also experience increased anxiety. There have been multiple mouse studies confirming the connection of pathogenic gut bacteria and stress behaviors via the gut–brain axis.

TESTING AND DIAGNOSIS

SIBO is typically diagnosed by a doctor through a combination of symptom review and SIBO breath test. Before ordering a SIBO test, some doctors will first rule out other possible causes, including gluten or dairy intolerance.

There are two types of substrates used in a SIBO test: lactulose or glucose. I recommend the lactulose test from the manufacturer QuinTron. Since glucose is easily digested, it only detects SIBO in the first few feet of the small intestine. A lactulose breath test can diagnose distal SIBO (where the SIBO is in the small intestine, in this case farther along; proximal SIBO is at the beginning of the small intestine), which tends to be more common.

The QuinTron SIBO test is a breath test that measures levels of gases—hydrogen and methane specifically—that are present in the breath when there is a bacterial overgrowth. A baseline sample is taken, a lactulose and water solution is consumed, and breath samples are taken every 20 minutes for three hours.

When reviewing your SIBO test with your doctor, keep the following in mind:

- Some doctors look at the first 90 minutes to diagnose, while others look at the first 120 minutes. The 120-minute mark is typically the transition between the small and large intestine. For people with very fast or very slow motility, the transition timing may be different.

- The recent Breath Test Consensus declared that a rise greater or equal to 20 ppm (parts per million) of hydrogen during the first 90 minutes of a lactulose or glucose breath test is considered positive, while a value greater or equal to 10 ppm of methane is considered positive. However, most doctors have their specific beliefs about test numbers due to their clinical experience. Some doctors or labs take into account numbers higher than 20 ppm for hydrogen or 10 ppm for methane at any point in the test—not looking at the *rise* only. Some doctors believe a SIBO test is positive for methane when methane is at 3 or above at any point in the 180-minute test if the person has symptoms of constipation. It's important to know how your doctor is reviewing your test and why.

- No matter what your SIBO numbers, it's also important to take your symptoms into account. Some people have relatively low numbers but have a multitude of symptoms. This can be for many reasons, such as associated issues or a person's sensitivity to symptoms.

- It's always vital to address the underlying cause—the possible reason you have SIBO—as that affects how quickly you heal. If you go through several different antibiotics and still have very little change in your numbers, it's likely you'll need to take a more in-depth look at your underlying cause or concurrent issues.

REASONS TO RETEST

1. Retesting after a round of antibiotics will indicate how you reacted to herbal or pharmaceutical antibiotics or an elemental diet (a very restricted therapeutic diet undertaken for two to three weeks as a treatment for SIBO) and how far your numbers were lowered. A larger drop in test numbers correlates with a greater effectiveness of treatment.

2. Retesting will determine if the overgrowth is gone. Some doctors will prescribe one round of antibiotics and assume the overgrowth is gone. Everyone reacts to treatments differently, so it's important to retest to see if the SIBO has actually been eradicated.

3. Seeing a negative test can be hopeful. There can be great relief in it. If you relapse, which some people do, it's also helpful to know you were able to get to a negative test. In the case of relapse, it may be time to take another look at your underlying cause or concurrent health issues.

WHEN NOT TO TEST

1. Lactulose produces laxative effects in many people, and, for some, it can have really negative health effects. Other people can't follow the prep outline without detrimental health ramifications. If this is your case, speak with your doctor about the possibility of treating the symptoms without a test result.

2. Many people have longer or even lifelong cases of SIBO or digestive distress. They come to an understanding of their symptoms and ongoing treatment, and the numbers don't necessarily matter. In fact, they may cause additional anxiety. Sometimes it can be helpful to take a break from testing or speak to an additional practitioner to look at your case in a different light. Don't give up, because there's always hope for improvement—both emotionally and physically. However, it's important to know and honor yourself, and, with your health practitioner, decide when testing is right for you.

Working with Your Doctor

It's of utmost importance to work with a knowledgeable and curious doctor whom you trust. Some doctors don't believe in SIBO, food intolerances, etc., or just don't know much about SIBO. Bring your doctor this book, your completed quiz, and the 2007 report "Small Intestinal Bacterial Overgrowth," published in the journal *Gastroenterology & Hepatology* (www.ncbi.nlm.nih.gov/pmc/articles/PMC3099351/), to start a conversation.

If you've been previously diagnosed with IBS, it's important to tell your doctor that 60 to 84 percent of IBS cases also involve SIBO. If this doesn't pique your doctor's interest, it might be time to seek help elsewhere. Check https://www.siboinfo.com/finding-a-doctor.html to find a doctor near your area. If there are no doctors in your area who are SIBO experts, you can consult with a doctor or nutritionist online. If you can only see a certain doctor because of your insurance, pick up the slack by doing your own research or finding another health practitioner who can help connect the dots.

For many people, healing from SIBO can be a long and challenging road. You may be sick and tired, frustrated, and overworked, yet you will always be one of your best resources because you know yourself better than anyone else ever will. Decide which pieces of your health support you need help with and which ones you can take care of on your own. Get used to conducting research and tracking symptoms, bowel movements, food choices, and moods. And know when to let that all go and focus on self-care. Develop your inner authority but be open to accepting help and support.

SIBO and Nutrition

Receiving a positive SIBO diagnosis can be frustrating and scary.

Yet for those who have been living with symptoms for years, it can be an exciting first step toward understanding their health issues and the start of healing.

In this chapter, we examine the process for eliminating SIBO, as well as how diet supports that. Choosing a SIBO diet can be confusing because there's not just one, but many, to choose from. The reason for this is that many practitioners have a different view of what will help people. Some diets are scientifically based and are often additionally based on the practitioner's clinical experience. Some work wonders for a specific person, but don't work for someone else. It's important to know as much as possible about your health picture when choosing a diet with the guidance of your health practitioner. Have you previously been diagnosed with IBS and/or do you react negatively to high-FODMAP foods? Do you have histamine intolerance, fructose malabsorption, or fat malabsorption? Do you tolerate starches? Depending on your intolerances and current health, it's important to start with a basic diet.

It's also important to remember there's no one-size-fits-all when it comes to nutrition, and a SIBO diet should be tailored to suit your needs.

In addition to reviewing popular diets, you'll learn about our 4-Week Meal Plan. I highlight types of foods to avoid, healing foods to add to your diet, and foods you'll need to assess—those that cause symptoms in some people but not all. We'll end by examining practices and supplements, in addition to diet, to reduce symptoms.

ELIMINATION

For most people, an antibiotic treatment or an elemental diet is necessary for eliminating SIBO. This might mean one or multiple rounds of antibiotics, depending on the size of overgrowth and response to treatment. Doctors often switch up protocols so they can ascertain which works best, as well as to avoid antibiotic resistance. For dosing and more information, visit SIBOinfo.com.

If you had higher breath test numbers, starting with the elemental diet can be helpful because, for some people, it reduces SIBO numbers more than pharmaceutical or herbal antibiotics. From a round of herbal or pharmaceutical antibiotics, numbers may go down anywhere between 15 and 40 points. From the elemental diet, numbers may go down 70 to 100 points. These ranges won't be true for everyone, and they also depend on concurrent issues and underlying causes.

During both treatment and the post-treatment healing phase, it can be helpful to adopt a SIBO diet, which will limit symptoms and support healing.

The following treatments are most often used for SIBO:

Antibiotics. These include rifaximin (Xifaxan) for all cases. For constipation, neomycin or metronidazole can be used in addition to rifaximin.

Herbal antibiotics. A 2014 study found that herbal antibiotics worked as well as rifaximin. Doctors often use a combination of herbals to address SIBO.

Elemental diet. This is a treatment by itself. It isn't a diet that one follows during other treatment. The elemental diet essentially starves bacteria to eradicate SIBO.

Prokinetics after treatment. A prokinetic is an herbal or pharmaceutical drug that stimulates motility of the gastrointestinal muscles by making contractions stronger or more frequent in support of the migrating motor complex (MMC), which produces a cleansing wave in the small intestine between meals. Most people take a prokinetic after a negative SIBO diagnosis to keep it from recurring. It can be taken for a couple of months and then removed slowly to see if motility remains healthy without it. It is generally considered a necessary part of making sure SIBO does not reoccur.

Homemade Elemental Diet

The homemade elemental diet was created by Dr. Allison Siebecker and is fully detailed on her informative website, SIBOinfo.com (see Resources, page 206).

The homemade elemental diet is fairly easy to make, but many people find it easier to purchase a premade elemental formula mix (which must be ordered through a practitioner.) Additionally, some people find the premade formula to be more palatable because the amino acids tend to have an off-putting taste. The benefits of the homemade formula are that it can be formulated to higher or lower carbohydrate levels, and it may be less expensive than some purchased options.

The elemental diet is followed for two weeks minimum to three weeks maximum. Some people will do the elemental diet for two weeks, take an in-person SIBO test with a 24-hour turnaround (not offered everywhere; see Resources [page 206] for Portland, OR, location), and follow the diet for a third week if they are still testing positive for SIBO. Another option is to follow the diet for three weeks and then take the SIBO test.

DIET

For the majority of people, a SIBO diet is meant to alleviate symptoms, not cure SIBO. Unfortunately, too many people cut out a significant variety of foods, experience unwanted weight loss, or have nutritional deficiencies. A SIBO diet should offer a diversity of nutrient-dense foods that will reduce symptoms. You'll likely still have some gastrointestinal symptoms, such as gas, burping, or bloating, and that isn't a major cause for alarm. It's inconvenient, sometimes even painful, but it is also our body's way of giving us information. Listen to your symptoms and work with them via SIBO treatment, diet, and self-care. For many people, symptoms change and lessen over time.

You'll find several popular diets listed here, as well as the one we'll use as our 4-Week Meal Plan. With SIBO, symptoms can be extremely varied, and one diet doesn't work for everyone. Long-term strict adherence to any restrictive diet can have negative physical, social, and emotional ramifications. Above all, continue to cultivate a positive relationship with food.

SIBO-SPECIFIC FOOD GUIDE (SSFG)

This diet, designed by Dr. Allison Siebecker, combines a low-FODMAP diet and Specific Carbohydrate Diet (SCD), and it is the most restrictive. Though it can be extremely helpful in symptom relief, many people don't eat foods outside of the "least fermentable" designation, contributing to the restrictiveness.

BI-PHASIC DIET (BPD)

This diet, designed by Dr. Nirala Jacobi, is based on Dr. Siebecker's SSFG diet and is updated with Dr. Jacobi's clinical experience. She uses a phased approach to introduce new foods over time.

SPECIFIC CARBOHYDRATE DIET (SCD)

This diet removes specific carbohydrates (polysaccharides, some oligosaccharides, disaccharides, and polyols) and has been shown effective in healing inflammatory bowel disease (IBD), but it has not been studied for SIBO. The legal/illegal food system can be very harmful, as it creates unrealistic expectations and fears. High-FODMAP foods are included in this diet and may still trigger symptoms in some people with SIBO.

3-Day Diet Diary

Name _____   Dates _____

   This diet diary will help you build a record of your eating habits over several days, for you and your health care practitioner. Simply eat and record your diet over three days, making sure one day is on a weekend. List the foods, drinks, ingredients, and amounts, including snacks. In the "Bowel Movements" column, list the time and quality of bowel movements. Under "Notes," list any symptoms such as mood, headaches, fatigue, bloating, etc., as well as any self-care for the day (i.e., exercise, meditation).

	Day 1	Day 2	Day 3
BREAKFAST			
LUNCH			
DINNER			
SNACKS			
NOTES			
BOWEL MOVEMENTS			

PALEO DIET

Eating paleo can be a positive change for people who feel healthier when eating organic meat, healthy fats, and selected fruits and vegetables. The paleo diet doesn't take high-FODMAP foods into account, so symptoms will persist for those who don't tolerate them. Unwanted weight loss may result for some who need to consume more calories from starchy vegetables and grains. Eating out on a paleo diet can be much easier because many restaurants have paleo options.

LOW FODMAPS (FERMENTABLE OLIGOSACCHARIDES, DISACCHARIDES, MONOSACCHARIDES, AND POLYOLS)

Removing high-FODMAP foods can be very helpful for people with SIBO, IBS, and leaky gut. Since people may be sensitive to some high-FODMAP foods but not others, it's possible you may not need to avoid all high-FODMAP foods. Long term, it is helpful to test FODMAPs by introducing specific high FODMAP foods and reincorporating the tolerated ones back into your diet. Many people don't tolerate many low-FODMAP foods such as grains, coconut, and various raw vegetables.

OUR MODIFIED LOW-FODMAP 4-WEEK MEAL PLAN

We will use low FODMAPs as the foundation of our 4-Week Meal Plan, and I highly recommend the Monash University Low FODMAP Diet app from Monash University for tracking low FODMAP amounts (see Resources, page 206). We will use a phased food introduction approach and focus on nutrient-dense, easily absorbed and digested foods to mitigate symptoms. The meal plan also includes an optional Calming Menu for those needing to start with simpler foods to calm unmanageable symptoms or for those who begin to experience a flare in the course of the meal plan that needs to be alleviated.

As the meal plan progresses, foods are added that some people will tolerate and others will not. During this time, it's important to chart your food intake, symptoms, mood, and bowel movements using a food diary (see page 17). If a food is clearly causing symptoms, remove it from the diet and make a substitution. You can also stay within Week 1 or Week 2 of the meal plan, or return to the Calming Menu, for a longer amount of time if more healing is needed, before adding greater food diversity.

HEALING FOODS

For most people with SIBO, food doesn't just provide energy or enjoyment; it also has a very direct connection to SIBO symptoms. This section reviews which foods are especially healing, any foods to avoid, and those foods that should be assessed to determine your individual tolerance.

FOODS TO AVOID

Low-quality food. Consider your food budget part of your health insurance. To incorporate more real, whole foods into your diet, review the Environmental Working Group's "Dirty Dozen" list (see Resources, page 206) of the most contaminated foods to help you select which organic fruits and vegetables to prioritize when shopping on a budget, as well as the Low-FODMAP Dirty Dozen and Clean 7 (see page 204) to help you select low-FODMAP organic fruits and vegetables specific to your needs.

Too many snacks. Because your body's migrating motor complex (MMC) performs a "cleansing wave" in the small intestine when you leave three to five hours between meals, only snack as needed to maintain a healthy weight so the body can do its good work to keep you healthy.

Processed or complicated foods. Eat simple meals with whole foods and few ingredients to help you assess whether foods in your diet contribute to your symptoms. Avoiding processed foods with additives, such as gums or food coloring, can make a big (positive!) difference.

Hard-to-digest foods. Since raw foods can be difficult to digest and contribute to your symptoms, eat smaller portions of them.

High-fiber foods. Many people are told to eat more fiber if they have constipation. With SIBO, eating a lot of fiber feeds bacteria, resulting in more symptoms. Introduce higher-fiber foods judiciously over time as you heal.

High-sugar foods. Though sugar isn't high-FODMAP, white table sugar is heavily processed and can have many ill effects on health. Most recipes in this book call for maple syrup, pasteurized clover honey, or Sucanat (an unprocessed form of cane sugar) in smaller amounts. It's fine to have a higher-sugar treat now and then, but it's best for your health to focus on eating healthy, whole, unprocessed foods.

Unhealthy fats. Avoid canola oil, corn oil, and partially hydrogenated vegetable oil, as they are often genetically modified and contain pesticides. See Foods to Eat (below) for healthy fat recommendations.

FOODS TO EAT

Low-FODMAP fruits and vegetables. Incorporate peeled, seeded, and well-cooked fruits and vegetables into easy-to-digest compotes, purées, soups, and stews. Introduce smaller portions of raw foods as you begin to heal.

Wild-caught salmon. Salmon has a high concentration of anti-inflammatory EPA and DHA omega-3 fatty acids, and its protein arrangement contains a mix of antioxidant and anti-inflammatory peptides. Limiting inflammation can reduce the risk of many chronic health conditions such as cancer, depression, and autoimmune diseases.

Grass-fed beef. This type of beef has a high amount of vitamins B_3 and B_{12}, protein, and the minerals zinc and iron. Beef liver can contain up to 100 times more nutrients than corresponding muscle meats. Vitamin B_3 (also known as niacin) is important in maintaining cardiovascular health. B_{12} is often low in people with SIBO, and it plays an essential role in red blood cell formation and nerve function.

Healthy fats. Safe and healthy oils and fats for cooking include organic ghee, coconut oil, beef tallow, or red palm oil. For light sautéing or no cooking, use extra-virgin olive oil, avocado oil, or organic grass-fed butter. Healthy fats contribute many benefits, including blood sugar regulation and vitamin absorption of fat-soluble vitamins A, D, E, and K, and they are anti-inflammatory, possibly lowering the risks of heart disease and stroke.

Fresh herbs and spices. Herbs and spices provide a variety of nutrients while also making food more attractive and tasty.

24-Hour Yogurt (page 84). Most store-bought yogurts have been fermented for seven to eight hours and include lactose. Fermenting yogurt for 24 hours removes the lactose and increases the probiotic levels.

FOODS TO ASSESS

The foods listed here are considered low-FODMAP but aren't tolerated by some people. Using your food diary as a guide, if you notice symptoms with a particular food, remove it from your diet and try another food instead.

Coconut. Some people do well with coconut, while it just doesn't sit well with others. It's helpful to figure out which side you're on.

Eggs. Many people tolerate eggs well, but for others, either the yolk or the white can be hard to digest.

Dairy. Some dairy is high-FODMAP because it contains lactose, a milk sugar. Even with lactose-free dairy, like hard aged cheeses, digesting casein or whey, the proteins contained in milk, may be an issue.

Nightshades. Potatoes, tomatoes, peppers, and eggplant are the most common nightshades. It is thought that nightshades cause inflammation, but there are few studies that back up that claim—and there are several studies that contradict the theory. Without removing nightshades haphazardly, it makes sense for everyone, especially those with autoimmune diseases, to further assess any personal connections between nightshade consumption and inflammation.

Nuts. Nuts can be hard to digest. Start by eating small amounts of nut milk or nut butter and then test nut flours or whole nuts.

Gluten. Some items that contain gluten are high-FODMAP and some are low-FODMAP. However, since many people don't tolerate gluten, it has been excluded from our 4-Week Meal Plan so it can be tested after one month.

Alcohol. Beer, gin, vodka, whiskey, red wine, sparkling wine, and white wine are all low-FODMAP. However, alcohol is often not well tolerated by people with IBS or SIBO. It's fine to have a drink at a party or while out to dinner, but sip judiciously and make a note in your diary of how you feel. If you overdo it, it will likely have more ramifications than it has previously.

Caffeine. Caffeine can be found in coffee, tea, and chocolate. Some people are very sensitive to it and find it irritates their gastrointestinal tract. Others feel it's helpful—both physically and emotionally. If you are very symptomatic, remove it for two weeks to see if your symptoms decrease.

SYMPTOM MITIGATION

Symptoms such as diarrhea, gas, bloating, or constipation can range from uncomfortable to debilitating. Along with changing your diet, addressing symptoms specifically with supplements or healing practices can make a big difference in symptom severity as you heal from SIBO. The supplements and practices listed here are ones that either I have personally tried and find helpful or that have worked for my clients. It's important to speak with a health care professional about your entire SIBO health picture before deciding on supplements or other symptom-mitigation practices.

CONSTIPATION

- Include healthy oils in your diet. Add 1 tablespoon of fish oil daily (you may need to work up to that), and make sure you eat healthy fats with each meal.

- Take magnesium glycinate (gentler), or magnesium oxide or citrate (more powerful but can be harsh). Start with about 240mg and increase the dose as needed.

- Try castor oil packs. Put the oil directly on your stomach, put on old pajamas or a T-shirt (they will get oily), and go to sleep. When you're awake and at home, put the oil on your stomach, put an old towel over it, and put a heating pad on top of that for an hour or more. Do this daily or nightly as needed.

- An Epsom salts bath can have a gentle laxative effect from the magnesium in the salts. Use at least 5 cups of Epsom salts in your hot bath and, if possible, soak until the water is lukewarm.

- Test a high-quality probiotic. In my experience, a probiotic supplement can help some people have more regular bowel movements, while for others it exacerbates symptoms. Some notice no difference at all. For those who don't notice a difference, I recommend trying a different probiotic. A 2014 study in the *Journal of Gastrointestinal and Liver Diseases* on the probiotic *L. reuteri* found it was helpful in increasing bowel movement frequency in adult patients with chronic constipation.

DIARRHEA

- Take activated charcoal. This should be for short-term use only, two to three days maximum in a flare situation. It will absorb water to decrease diarrhea, but it will also absorb nutrients and can cause constipation.

- If you're having an episode of diarrhea, replenish fluids with an electrolyte drink. Store-bought drinks aren't always optimal because they contain food coloring and sugar. Try my Homemade Electrolyte Drink (page 177) instead.

- Test a high-quality probiotic. A 2012 study on the probiotic *Saccharomyces boulardii* showed it to be helpful for those with a diarrhea symptom picture.

MULTIPLE SYMPTOMS

- Remove or limit potentially offending foods such as raw vegetables, including salads, smoothies with high concentrations of raw veggies or fruit, and high-FODMAP or fiber-rich foods. Following the diet outlined in this book will make a difference in the symptom picture of most people.

- Try Iberogast, an herbal formula that can be taken a couple of ways. For bloating, constipation, nausea, a feeling of uncomfortable fullness, and gas, I recommend drinking 20 to 30 drops in ½ cup of warm water with meals. If you tend to feel more symptoms around bedtime and when you wake up, take 20 to 30 drops in ½ cup of warm water at night and 20 to 30 drops in ½ cup of warm water in the morning.

- For diarrhea, bloating, or gas, take digestive enzymes, such as Klaire Labs Vital-Zymes or SIBB-Zymes, with every meal. If your digestion is compromised, enzymes can be a key part of digestive support.

- Stress can increase symptoms and affect overall health. Try supportive practices, like meditation, breath work, and gratitude, to relieve stress and help return you to the present moment.

Rebuild and Plan for the Month Ahead

Major life changes are typically a series of smaller choices and actions.

Although having SIBO isn't a choice anyone would make, beginning the healing process is an opportunity that can begin right away. Part of the process is laying the groundwork for the meal plan and being able to maintain a SIBO-friendly diet that works for you.

Making a commitment to your health includes following and maintaining this 4-Week Meal Plan, which may mean more preparation and cooking than you're used to. Likely, you will be trying new foods and removing some foods from your diet. To help you, the recipes included here are health supporting, delicious, and easy to prepare. There may be some challenges during the process, but the takeaway will likely be more self-knowledge, decreased symptoms, and new hope for healing.

You've probably been experiencing symptoms for longer than you'd like to admit and have wondered when you'd ever start feeling like your old self again. This meal plan has been created specifically for those with leaky gut, IBS, and SIBO, so you can begin to take control of and regain your health.

When you're ready, begin the process by making a commitment to rebuilding your health and your life. You can do this. I can help.

REBUILD YOUR KITCHEN

The first place to start is in the kitchen. Is yours ready to support your new approach to food? People often describe cleaning, organizing, and removing items they don't need as cathartic. It's a chance to begin again—in a more organized and deliberate way.

In this chapter, we embark on the process of commencing the meal plan by preparing the pantry and kitchen. During this time, you'll learn which grocery items are must-haves and which are important to remove.

As you'll likely be spending more time in your kitchen, we'll review kitchen equipment to help it function seamlessly. In turn, cooking will become easier and more approachable. Beginning this process by revamping your kitchen may help you feel lighter and more organized, and it is certainly one of the necessary first steps in healing from SIBO.

THE PANTRY

There are certain items you won't need in your pantry during your healing process. Remove garlic powder and fresh garlic, and replace it with low-FODMAP garlic oil. Replace canola and vegetable oils with coconut oil, ghee, organic grass-fed butter, and avocado and extra-virgin olive oils. Buy organics when possible. The following lists detail the essential items to stock in your pantry so you can easily be prepared to cook the recipes in this book.

A note about clover honey: Dr. Siebecker has researched clover honey and found it to have a 50/50 glucose to fructose level, making it low-FODMAP. Assess various sweeteners to see which you tolerate best.

Fresh and Dried Herbs and Spices

- Cardamom, ground
- Cinnamon, ground and sticks
- Cumin, ground
- Curry powder
- Ginger, ground and fresh
- Italian seasoning, without garlic
- Oregano, dried and fresh
- Peppercorns, for freshly ground pepper
- Sea salt
- Turmeric, ground and fresh

Canned and Bottled Items

- Mayonnaise, garlic-free and without gums
- Mustard, garlic-free and onion-free
- Tomato paste, organic

Oils and Vinegars

- Oils: avocado, coconut, garlic (low-FODMAP), extra-virgin olive, MCT
- Vinegars: apple cider, aged balsamic, red wine, white wine

- Flours: almond
- Quinoa
- White rice
- White rice noodles

Fresh Fruits and Vegetables

- Bananas
- Citrus fruits: lemons, limes, oranges
- Tomatoes
- Sweet potatoes
- White potatoes, organic

Sweeteners

- Clover honey, pasteurized
- Maple syrup
- Whole cane sugar, such as Sucanat

Other Pantry Items

- Almond butter
- Baking soda
- Bone broth, low-FODMAP or homemade
- Chocolate, dark (70 percent cacao or higher)
- Coconut aminos
- Coconut, dried, unsweetened
- Coconut cream
- Coffee
- Collagen hydrolysate (Great Lakes or Vital Proteins brand)
- Gelatin powder, grass-fed (Great Lakes brand)
- Tea, herbal, black, or green
- Vanilla extract

THE REFRIGERATOR

To get started, replace regular cow's milk with lactose-free dairy or coconut milk, almond milk, or other nut milks. Gums in most commercial milks bother some people but not all. Coconut milk can be made from dry coconut as needed (see Blueberry-Coconut Milk variation tip, page 176).

Nightshades, the family of vegetables that includes tomatoes, potatoes, peppers, paprika, chili powder, and eggplant, are included in some of these lists and recipes. Nightshades may cause inflammation in some people but not all. If you suspect an inflammatory response to eating nightshades, remove them and reintroduce one to see if you still notice a negative symptom correlation.

For proteins, I always recommend organic, free-range, grass-fed meats. Meat from healthy animals is very important because animals are on the top of the food chain, and if they are exposed to toxins via antibiotics or illness, GMO grains and pesticides, these are then passed on to the person eating it. Eating fattier cuts of meat will help those who are underweight or often hungry. Many people with SIBO tend to have malabsorption issues, so eating healthy oils and fattier meats can help with satiation.

Check your refrigerator and stock up on the following items as needed.

Dairy

- 24-Hour Yogurt (page 84)
- Butter, organic grass-fed, or ghee

Liquids

- Milk of choice, selecting from coconut, almond or other nuts, lactose-free dairy—free of gums, if possible

Proteins

- Bacon
- Beef, ground and a variety of cuts
- Chicken, organic, whole, thighs, wings, and livers
- Deli meat, organic, without garlic
- Eggs, organic, pastured
- Pork, ground and a variety of cuts
- Seafood, cod, mahi-mahi, salmon, shrimp, and swordfish

Produce

- Bell peppers
- Broccoli
- Carrots
- Chives, fresh
- Cilantro, fresh
- Eggplant
- Green beans
- Kale
- Lettuce, soft
- Mint, fresh
- Olives, fresh or canned or jarred, without garlic
- Parsley, fresh
- Sage, fresh
- Scallions
- Spinach
- Zucchini

THE FREEZER

As you'll be eating less processed food from here on out, you'll have more room in your freezer for leftovers for meals in a hurry. Almond flours (from your pantry list, page 27) are best kept in the freezer if not used frequently.

If you enjoy smoothies, sauté spinach with a little oil, divide it among an ice cube tray, add your desired milk, and freeze—instant smoothie ice cubes. Once frozen, remove them from the tray and keep in airtight freezer-safe containers (preferably not plastic). Frozen fruit can be also used for smoothies.

If you buy frozen meat or seafood (from your pantry list, see above) in bulk (it can be far less expensive that way), you'll have it on hand when you need it.

- Beef marrow bones for bone broth
- Beef stew meat for bone broth
- Frozen bone broth
- Frozen fruit: peeled banana chunks, blueberries, strawberries
- Frozen meals or meal components

10 SIBO Diet Tips for Cooking and Enjoying Food

1. **Be patient with yourself.** Making big changes can feel overwhelming at first. Give yourself time to adjust and you'll be ready before you know it.

2. **Set a beautiful table.** Bring out the nice dishes and napkins. Set out flowers. Incorporate small touches to make every meal special.

3. **Rethink family meals.** Instead of a separate meal just for you, make something the entire family can add on to. For example, if you've made meat loaf and a carrot purée for yourself, family members can have a meat loaf sandwich—or enjoy what you're eating.

4. **Slow down.** Whenever possible, start the digestion process by smelling your food as it cooks. Turn off the TV. Enjoy good conversation and relax.

5. **Express gratitude.** Before you start eating, reflect on your day and notice one thing that touched you. Studies show that gratitude is linked to greater physical and emotional health.

6. **Take shortcuts.** Buy precut vegetables and fruits, or premade items like a roasted chicken.

7. **Avoid adding guilt and fear to your diet.** Don't use guilt and fear as motivational tools. The diet is supposed to work for you—you don't work for the diet.

8. **Try batch cooking.** Make larger batches of food and freeze portions to eat later. Take frozen foods for lunch or pull out frozen items for dinner.

9. **Keep trying.** Many people are hyperaware of their symptoms and fear trying new foods. Symptoms after food testing are your body's way of offering feedback. While manageable symptoms are the goal, it's typically unrealistic to expect not to have any at all.

10. **Accept help.** You may be cooking more than you have in the past. Ask for help from family or friends, or consider hiring a short-term personal chef, if possible. But remember, the recipes here are easy, accessible, and delicious—all designed to support your health goals.

COOKING EQUIPMENT

If you're used to cooking at home, you'll likely already have many items listed here. If not, don't dismay. You can collect new items over time, and there are always work-arounds for equipment you may not have. However, I'll warn you, once you get some of these time-saving items you'll wonder how you ever lived without them!

When at all possible, I limit plastic storage containers in the kitchen, so I recommend glass for storage instead.

Equipment essentials

- Baking sheets
- Blender
- Bowl scraper
- Can opener
- Cupcake pan
- Cutting board
- Food processor
- Glass canning jars for food and drink storage, variety of sizes
- Ice cube tray
- Knives, including a good chef's knife and paring knife
- Ladle
- Large pot or Dutch oven
- Loaf pan
- Measuring cups
- Measuring spoons
- Metal cooling rack
- Mixing bowls, various sizes
- Peeler
- Rectangular baking pan
- Skillet or sauté pan
- Spatula
- Tongs
- Whisk
- Wooden spoons

Nice-to-have equipment

- Funnel
- Immersion blender
- Juicer
- Large soup pot or stockpot
- Nut milk bag
- Pressure cooker, such as the Instant Pot
- Silicone baking sheet liners
- Silicone cupcake liners
- Silicone gummy molds
- Slow cooker
- Spiralizer

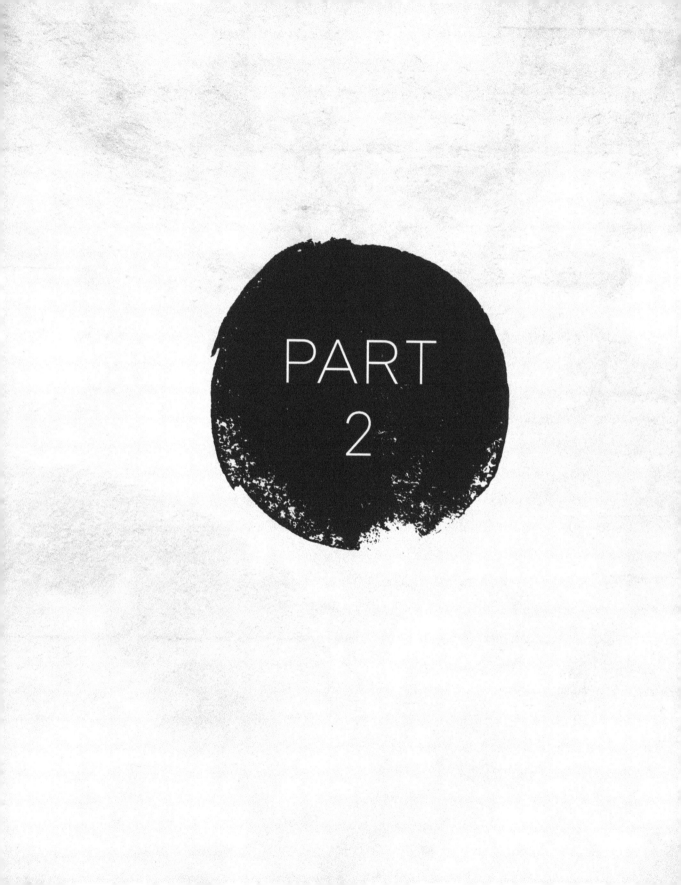

PART

2

The 4-Week Meal Plan

his 4-Week Meal Plan, with an optional preplan Calming Menu, has been constructed for symptom relief, nutrient density, and ease of use. For breakfast and lunch, leftovers are incorporated from previous meals as well as prepared-in-advance items for when you're ready to grab and go.

The Calming Menu is intended for those who have unmanageable symptoms and need first to calm their system. The recipes are very basic and will be well tolerated by most people.

For those who use the Calming Menu as the first week, you will then move on to Week 1 and only use the first three weeks of the meal plan.

In Week 1, the foods are meant to be easily digestible with simple and straightforward recipes. They include softer foods such as soups and purées. Rice is introduced here, but all other grains and higher-starch foods are avoided for the first week.

In Week 2, lactose-free dairy, alternative milks, and white and sweet potatoes are added.

During Week 3, side salads and dark chocolate are added.

In Week 4, we add nuts, coconut, and quinoa.

After the meal plan, chapter 5 offers practical tips and information for moving beyond the four weeks. We've got you covered.

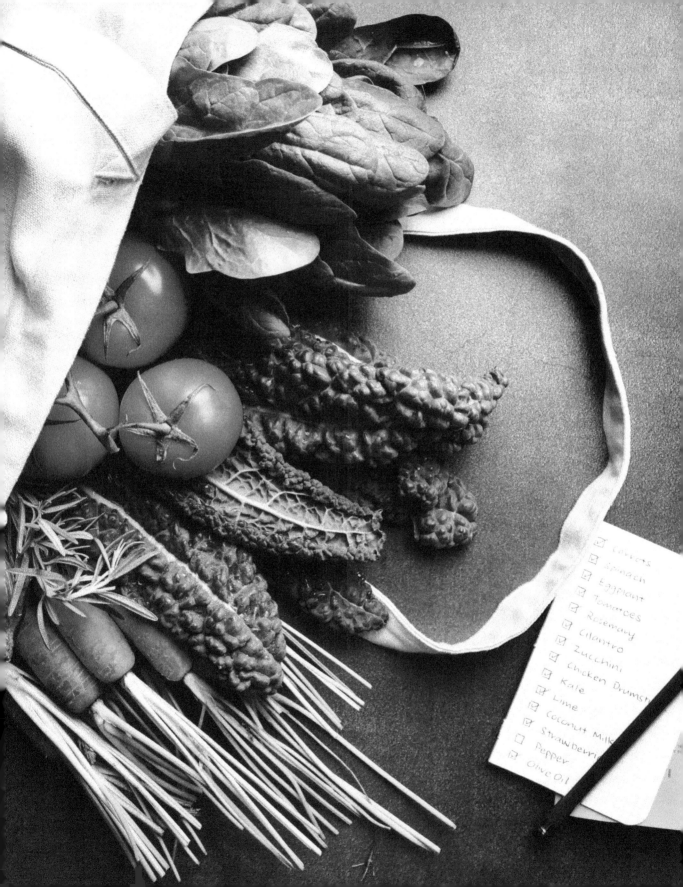

- ☑ Carrots
- ☐ Spinach
- ☑ Eggplant
- ☑ Tomatoes
- ☑ Rosemary
- ☑ Cilantro
- ☑ Zucchini
- ☑ Chicken Drumst
- ☑ Kale
- ☑ Lime
- ☑ Coconut Milk
- ☐ Strawberri
- ☑ Pepper
- ☑ Olive Oil

The Plan

It's here . . . the time to start
your healing journey.

As you begin this meal plan, listen to your body's feedback in the form of symptoms (or their improvement). If you're progressing through the weeks with manageable symptoms, that's great. If not, you may need to back up to the Calming Menu, or to Week 1 or Week 2, and stay there until more healing occurs. No matter what, keep a food diary (see page 17) and start this meal plan with a sense of curiosity and kindness toward yourself. Remember, you are doing this for you!

Meal Plan Troubleshooting 101

The following tips can help you manage the unexpected or uncomfortable side effects during your 4-Week Meal Plan. However, if you are in a flare state or are having unmanageable symptoms, consult your health care practitioner.

Cramping or bowel grumbling after eating. Eat slowly and chew your food thoroughly. Try taking a digestive enzyme at the beginning of your meal to support digestion. Focus more on soups, purées, and other easier-to-digest foods.

Can't digest meat. Try drinking 1 teaspoon of apple cider vinegar mixed with 1 cup of water before each meal. Also consider a digestive enzyme that includes hydrochloric acid (see Resources, page 206).

Reacting to eggs. Eggs are included in the menu because of their versatility and nutrient density. If you don't tolerate them, prepare other recipes denoted as Week 1+, meaning you can eat them during the first week or later during the 4-week plan.

Reacting to vegetables. Start with vegetables you know you tolerate and slowly add more. Experiment with the amount and frequency of different vegetables to see what you tolerate best. You can also eat basic cooked meats without sauces or multiple ingredients to see if that eases your symptoms.

Reacting to rice. You may not be able to process any starchy grains, or it could just be that rice doesn't work for you right now. Add a different starch, like peeled white potatoes. If that doesn't work, remove rice or potatoes for a week or two and add one back to see if you still have symptoms.

Always hungry. You may have malabsorption issues. If this is the case, you're not able to absorb all the nutrients your body needs, so you're constantly hungry, needing extra calories. If you experience unwanted weight loss, make sure you're eating fat and carbohydrate combinations and drinking homemade beverages like Ginger Limeade (page 174) or Blueberry-Coconut Milk (page 176) with each meal for additional calories.

Getting full too quickly. Chew your food thoroughly and slowly. Take a digestive enzyme and 1 teaspoon of apple cider vinegar mixed with 1 cup of water before meals. Until the fullness changes, you may need to eat more frequent, smaller meals. This isn't ideal because it's preferable to support the migrating motor complex by leaving three to five hours between meals. However, it may be helpful in the short term until the situation changes.

General nausea. Try drinking ginger tea when you're nauseous and take a digestive enzyme before meals.

Nausea from eating fat. You may have fat malabsorption issues. Eat smaller amounts of fat less frequently until you can ascertain what amount works for you. Try to build up the amount again over time.

Experiencing increased symptoms after the first week of the meal plan. If you start having more symptoms later in the meal plan, it's likely you don't tolerate a new item. If you suspect there's a particular food you're not tolerating, remove it for a week or two and reintroduce it. It's definitely okay to stay in Week 1 or 2 of the meal plan for the entire four weeks.

Reacting to leftovers, bone broth, or vinegars. This could possibly be a histamine intolerance. Histamine intolerance symptoms vary greatly and may include itching, skin rash, hives, sore throat, or headaches. Remove any high-histamine items, including vinegars, leftovers, aged cheeses, cured meats, and fermented foods, from your menu for a week to see if your symptoms change.

Also, freeze and reheat any leftovers instead of leaving them in the refrigerator. When leftovers are left in the refrigerator, they become higher in histamines. Freezing them halts this process. So, if you have histamine intolerance, it's better to freeze and reheat meals than leave them in the refrigerator for a couple of days.

CALMING MENU

This optional week is the place to start the plan if you are experiencing unmanage-able symptoms, persistent diarrhea, or overwhelming food sensitivities, before diving into the 4-Week Meal Plan.

This menu includes meats, rice, and generally well-tolerated vegetables including carrots, green beans, spinach, and zucchini. The vegetables are mostly featured in soups and purées because those foods are hydrating and easy to digest. Eggs are included on the menu for diversity and ease, but not everyone tolerates them. If there is something on this menu you do not tolerate, switch it out for another known tolerated food or remove it altogether.

As you work through this menu, if possible, make sure each meal includes protein, carbohydrates in the form of vegetables or rice, and healthy fats. This menu is here to help you get started and calm symptoms, but use it as a tool to customize to your individual needs. If you have a flare or experience new unmanageable symptoms as you progress from Week 1 to Week 4, this is the place to return until you are once again at a neutral point as you work toward greater healing. The Calming Menu can be used for just a couple of days or longer, as needed. To ensure nutrient diversity, though, it's important to move past the Calming Menu when possible.

If your symptoms are not as severe and you can eat a wider variety of foods, start directly with the Week 1 Meal Plan (see page 44).

CALMING MENU SHOPPING LIST

Canned and Bottled Items

☐ Coconut water, without added sugar or juices (1 cup)

Dairy and Eggs

☐ Butter, organic grass-fed, or ghee (1 pound)
☐ Eggs, pastured (2 dozen large)

Meat and Poultry

☐ Bacon (3 slices)
☐ Chicken, boneless, skinless organic breasts (1 pound)
☐ Chicken, rotisserie (seasoned with salt and pepper only) or whole organic, 1 (2 or 3 pounds)
☐ Lamb chops, grass-fed organic (8 baby chops)
☐ Pork chops, thick-cut, bone-in, 2 (5 ounces each)
☐ Steak, grass-fed boneless sirloin, rib eye, or similar (1½ pounds)

Seafood

- ☐ White fish, such as cod or sole (2 or 3 pounds)

Pantry Items

- ☐ Apple cider vinegar
- ☐ Broth, 1 of the following:
  - • 1 batch of Low-FODMAP Vegetable Broth (page 90)
  - • 8 to 12 cups of low-FODMAP chicken or beef broth (see Resources, page 206)
  - • 2 batches of Pressure Cooker Bone Broth (page 92)
- ☐ Clover honey, pasteurized, or maple syrup
- ☐ Coconut oil, optional
- ☐ Extra-virgin olive oil
- ☐ Garlic oil
- ☐ Peppercorns
- ☐ Sea salt
- ☐ Tea, green, honeybush, rooibos, or peppermint
- ☐ White rice
- ☐ White rice noodles, made with white rice or white rice flour and water only, 8-ounce packages (2)

Produce

- ☐ Avocado (1)
- ☐ Carrots or baby carrots (5 pounds)
- ☐ Celery, organic (1 stalk)
- ☐ Ginger, fresh (8-inch piece)
- ☐ Green beans (½ pound)
- ☐ Lemons, nonorganic (5) and organic (1)
- ☐ Parsley, fresh (1 large bunch)
- ☐ Rosemary, fresh (1 bunch)
- ☐ Scallions (1 bunch)
- ☐ Spinach, fresh, prewashed organic (5 cups)
- ☐ Thyme, fresh (1 small bunch)
- ☐ Tomato, organic (1)
- ☐ Turmeric, fresh (3-inch piece)
- ☐ Zucchini (10 small or 7 medium)

Calming Menu Meal Prep

Use these tips to help you plan your kitchen and cooking time as you ease into your new way of thinking about food.

WEEKEND BULK COOKING

- Purchase rotisserie chicken (seasoned with salt and pepper only) or roast a whole organic chicken.
- Make a double batch of Pressure Cooker Bone Broth (page 92) or purchase low-FODMAP bone broth (see Resources, page 206).
- Make Detoxifying Vegetable Soup (page 91).
- Make Puréed Zucchini Soup (page 93).
- Make Cinnamon Rice (page 79).
- Make Breakfast Egg Muffins (page 80) and freeze some for later.
- Make Slow Cooker Roast Beef (page 144) on Sunday and save until Monday night for dinner, or start on Monday morning for Monday night.

EASY WEEKDAY COOKING

- Weeknight dinners are made nightly and designed to be quick and simple.
- Homemade Electrolyte Drink (page 177) can be prepared over the weekend or on Monday night.
- Make Ginger-Turmeric Tea (page 170) on Saturday or Sunday morning.

- Eat the amount that is right for you. Calorie intake will vary by person.
- Hardboiled eggs are an easily portable breakfast or snack and can be purchased precooked.
- Buy precut vegetables to save time.
- If you favor a paleo or grain-free diet, don't add rice when following the Calming Menu. However, if you are experiencing unwanted weight loss, fatigue, or tend to be hungry all the time, adding grains like rice may be helpful. Substitute a different grain you tolerate as desired.
- You'll notice some "dinner"-type items like soup or leftovers incorporated into breakfast for convenience and nutrition. Soup for breakfast is easy to take on the go and a healthy start to the day.
- If you need to switch out a recipe because you don't like or tolerate one listed, choose one denoted as "Calming Menu+," meaning it is appropriate for both the Calming Menu and later weeks of the diet.
- Water isn't noted on the diet—stay hydrated; it affects your digestion.
- All the recipes are designed to be low FODMAP in one serving. If you are going to eat more than one serving at a meal, check to make sure the ingredients are low FODMAP in the amount you're eating, particularly for recipes that include sweet potatoes or green beans.

Calming Menu

	Monday	Tuesday	Wednesday	
BREAKFAST	Pressure Cooker Bone Broth (page 92) 2 eggs, fried or hardboiled Cinnamon Rice (page 79)	Homemade Electrolyte Drink (page 177) 3 bacon slices Detoxifying Vegetable Soup (page 91)	Pressure Cooker Bone Broth (page 92) Breakfast Egg Muffins (page 80)	
LUNCH	Detoxifying Vegetable Soup (page 91) Simple Roast Chicken (page 132)	Puréed Zucchini Soup (page 93) Slow Cooker Roast Beef (page 144) Buttery Rice Noodles (page 122)	Basic Carrot Soup (page 94) Simple Roast Chicken (page 132) Basic White Rice (page 120)	
DINNER	Slow Cooker Roast Beef (page 144) Buttery Rice Noodles (page 122)	Basic Carrot Soup (page 94) Easy Baked White Fish (page 160) Basic White Rice (page 120)	Detoxifying Vegetable Soup (page 91) Poached Chicken Breast (page 133) Buttery Rice Noodles (page 122)	
DESSERTS OR SNACKS	Puréed Zucchini Soup (page 93)	Pressure Cooker Bone Broth (page 92)	Leftover Buttery Rice Noodles or Breakfast Egg Muffins (page 80)	

Thursday	Friday	Saturday	Sunday
Homemade Electrolyte Drink (page 177) Sautéed Spinach (page 107) Cinnamon Rice (page 79)	Pressure Cooker Bone Broth (page 92) Breakfast Egg Muffins (page 80) Basic Carrot Soup (page 94)	Pork Chops with Chimichurri Sauce (page 146) Basic Carrot Soup (page 94) Cinnamon Rice (page 79)	Ginger-Turmeric Tea (page 170) Savory Egg Scramble (page 78)
Detoxifying Vegetable Soup (page 91) Slow Cooker Roast Beef (page 144)	Puréed Zucchini Soup (page 93) Poached Chicken Breast (page 133)	Detoxifying Vegetable Soup (page 91) Poached Chicken Breast (page 133)	Rosemary Lamb Chops (page 147) Carrot-Ginger Purée (page 106)
Puréed Zucchini Soup (page 93) Easy Baked White Fish (page 160) Basic White Rice (page 120)	Detoxifying Vegetable Soup (page 91) Pork Chops with Chimichurri Sauce (page 146) Buttery Rice Noodles (page 122)	Rosemary Lamb Chops (page 147) Carrot-Ginger Purée (page 106) Buttery Rice Noodles (page 122)	Simple Steak (page 145) Basic White Rice (page 120)
Pressure Cooker Bone Broth (page 92)	Leftover Breakfast Egg Muffins or Detoxifying Vegetable Soup (page 91)	Pressure Cooker Bone Broth (page 92)	Hardboiled egg or Pressure Cooker Bone Broth (page 92)

WEEK 1

Starting something new can be scary. In the case of this meal plan, it's set up to be uncomplicated and user-friendly. You might be worried, however, about the possibility of introducing new foods or about the amount of time you'll need to spend cooking. Be assured: You are empowering yourself and investing in your health and well-being. As you begin this one-month meal plan, try to give yourself extra time for cooking, using your diet diary, and taking time to relax.

It's challenging to have chronic digestive issues, and many people tend to be on high alert as a result. That's why it's so important, in addition to following the meal plan, to take time during these four weeks to incorporate other activities that help you feel whole, like meditation, yoga, walking, or writing. This meal plan should be a key component to restoring your health, and it's part of your journey to find multiple ways to continue to heal.

WEEK 1 SHOPPING LIST

Canned and Bottled Items

- ☐ Mayonnaise (1 tablespoon)
- ☐ Mustard, without garlic or other high-FODMAP additives (1 tablespoon)
- ☐ Tomato paste, organic, small can (1)

Dairy and Eggs

- ☐ Butter, organic grass-fed, or ghee (1 pound)
- ☐ Eggs, pastured (2 dozen large)
- ☐ Yogurt, 1 of the following:
  - • 1 jar of premade 24-hour yogurt (White Mountain Bulgarian brand)
  - • 1 batch of 24-Hour Yogurt (page 84)

Meat and Poultry

- ☐ Bacon (2 pounds)
- ☐ Beef, ground, grass-fed (1 pound)
- ☐ Chicken, organic skins (6) and organic livers (½ pound)
- ☐ Chicken, rotisserie (seasoned with salt and pepper only) or whole organic, 1 (2 or 3 pounds)
- ☐ Deli meat, organic (6 slices)
- ☐ Flank steak, grass-fed (1 or 2 pounds)
- ☐ Pancetta, sliced (8 ounces)
- ☐ Pork, ground (1 pound)
- ☐ Pork chops, thick-cut, bone-in, 2 (5 ounces each)
- ☐ Pork shoulder or butt (2 pounds)
- ☐ Pork tenderloins, 2 (about 2 pounds)

Seafood

☐ Cod or sole (2 to 3 pounds)

☐ Salmon, 5-ounce fillets (2)

Pantry Items

☐ Aged balsamic vinegar

☐ Apple cider vinegar

☐ Avocado oil

☐ Broth, 1 of the following:
- 1 batch of Low-FODMAP Vegetable Broth (page 90)
- 8 to 12 cups of low-FODMAP chicken or beef broth (see Resources, page 206)
- 2 batches of Pressure Cooker Bone Broth (page 92)

☐ Clover honey, pasteurized

☐ Coconut aminos

☐ Coconut oil

☐ Extra-virgin olive oil

☐ Garlic oil

☐ Gelatin powder, grass-fed (Great Lakes brand)

☐ Maple syrup

☐ Red wine vinegar

☐ White rice

☐ White rice noodles, made with white rice or white rice flour and water only, 8-ounce package (1)

Produce

☐ Avocado, small (1)

☐ Banana (1)

☐ Carrots (3 pounds; prewashed, peeled baby carrots are easiest)

☐ Celery, organic (1 bunch)

☐ Chives, fresh (2 bunches)

☐ Eggplant (1 medium and 2 small)

☐ Ginger, fresh (10-inch piece)

☐ Green beans (2 pounds)

☐ Lemons (8)

☐ Limes, nonorganic (11) and organic (2)

☐ Microgreens, small package (1)

☐ Oranges, organic (2)

☐ Parsley, fresh (1 bunch)

☐ Pineapple, fresh chunks (3 cups)

☐ Rosemary, fresh (1 bunch)

☐ Scallions (2 bunches)

☐ Spinach, fresh, prewashed organic (6 cups)

☐ Thyme, fresh (1 bunch)

☐ Tomatoes, organic regular (2) and organic plum (4 large)

☐ Turmeric, fresh (3-inch piece)

☐ Zucchini, (3 large and 1 small)

Week 1 Meal Prep

Meal prep is listed as to what can be done over the weekend versus during the week, but you decide what's best for you. Some people may want to make and freeze all of their soup or breakfast muffins for a month and then defrost them to use during the week, while for others it will be easier to do the meal prep as listed. It's always good to have a couple of extra things in the freezer in case you don't like or tolerate something on the menu. If you find yourself in a pinch without prepared food, an organic roasted chicken with just salt and pepper can be a lifesaver. It will take a bit of planning, but you can do this, and the benefits will be well worth it.

WEEKEND BULK COOKING

- Purchase rotisserie chicken (seasoned with salt and pepper only) or roast a whole chicken.
- Make Pressure Cooker Bone Broth (page 92) or purchase low-FODMAP bone broth (see Resources, page 206).
- Make Detoxifying Vegetable Soup (page 91).
- Make Breakfast Egg Muffins (page 80) and freeze some for later.
- Make Ginger-Turmeric Tea (page 170).
- Make Lime Curd (page 182). This is an optional snack, so if you don't have time to make it, substitute bone broth, hardboiled eggs, or Sautéed Banana (page 171).

EASY WEEKDAY COOKING

- Weeknight dinners are made nightly and designed to be quick and simple.
- Moroccan Carrot Soup (page 96) and Chicken and Rice Soup (page 95) can be made over the weekend or on a weeknight.
- Marinate flank steak overnight on Tuesday for a Wednesday dinner.
- Make the Slow Cooker Pork and Pineapple (page 149) on Friday night or Saturday morning.
- Make Sour Gummies (page 173) on a weeknight or Saturday. If you have kids, it's a great shared activity.

- Double or halve recipes depending on leftovers used later in the week and if you're eating with other people.
- Eat the amount that is right for you. Calorie intake will vary by person.
- Hardboiled eggs are an easily portable breakfast or snack and can be purchased precooked.
- Buy precut vegetables to save time.
- If you favor a paleo or grain-free diet, don't add rice this first week. However, if you are experiencing unwanted weight loss, fatigue, or tend to be hungry all the time, adding grains like rice may be helpful.
- You'll notice some "dinner"-type items like soup or leftovers incorporated into breakfast for convenience and nutrition. Soup for breakfast is easy to take on the go and is a healthy start to the day.
- If you need to switch out a recipe because you don't like or tolerate one listed, choose one denoted by Calming Menu+ or Week 1+, meaning it is appropriate for the Calming Menu or first week of the diet.
- Water isn't noted on the diet—stay hydrated; it affects your digestion.
- All the recipes are designed to be low FODMAP in one serving. If you are going to eat more than one serving at a meal, check to make sure the ingredients are low FODMAP in the amount you're eating, particularly for recipes that include sweet potatoes or green beans.

Week 1 Menu

	Monday	Tuesday	Wednesday	
BREAKFAST	Pressure Cooker Bone Broth (page 92) Breakfast Egg Muffins (page 80)	Detoxifying Vegetable Soup (page 91) 3 bacon slices	Pressure Cooker Bone Broth (page 92) Breakfast Egg Muffins (page 80)	
LUNCH	Detoxifying Vegetable Soup (page 91) Deli Meat Roll-Ups (page 134)	Chicken and Rice Soup (page 95) Carrot-Ginger Purée (page 106)	Pancetta-Wrapped Pork Tenderloin (page 148) Carrot-Ginger Purée (page 106)	
DINNER	Simple Roast Chicken (page 132) Carrot-Ginger Purée (page 106) Herbed Rice (page 121)	Pancetta-Wrapped Pork Tenderloin (page 148) Herbed Rice (page 121)	Detoxifying Vegetable Soup (page 91) Easy Flank Steak (page 151) Herbed Rice (page 121)	
DESSERTS OR SNACKS	Sautéed Banana (page 171)	Pressure Cooker Bone Broth (page 92)	Lime Curd (page 182)	

Thursday	Friday	Saturday	Sunday
Ginger-Turmeric Tea (page 170) Pancetta-Wrapped Pork Tenderloin (page 148) Sautéed Spinach (page 107)	Pressure Cooker Bone Broth (page 92) Fried or hardboiled egg Roasted Vegetables with Bacon (page 109)	Detoxifying Vegetable Soup (page 91) Pork Chops with Chimichurri Sauce (page 146)	Ginger-Turmeric Tea (page 170) Moroccan Carrot Soup (page 96) Savory Egg Scramble (page 78)
Ginger Limeade (page 174) Chicken and Rice Soup (page 95)	Leftover Easy Flank Steak Balsamic Green Beans (page 111)	Meat Loaf with Liver (page 150) Roasted Vegetables with Bacon (page 109)	Slow Cooker Pork and Pineapple (page 149) Sautéed Spinach (page 107)
Pressure Cooker Bone Broth (page 92) Baked Eggplant (page 110) Honey-Mustard Salmon (page 162)	Pork Chops with Chimichurri Sauce (page 146) Carrot-Ginger Purée (page 106)	Moroccan Carrot Soup (page 96) Slow Cooker Pork and Pineapple (page 149)	Easy Baked White Fish (page 160) Buttery Rice Noodles (page 122)
Chicken Chips (page 172)	Lime Curd (page 182)	Pressure Cooker Bone Broth (page 92)	Sour Gummies (page 173)

WEEK 2

Congratulations on finishing the Week 1 Meal Plan! Review your food diary to remind yourself of any symptoms, bowel movements, and mood changes, as well as your self-care and the results from it. This will not only help with connecting food intolerances to symptoms but can give you a better picture of your overall health. This past week, you may have noticed fewer symptoms since adopting this low-FODMAP diet. If you haven't noticed any symptom decrease at all, keep with it another week. If your system was in a very inflamed state, it may take a couple weeks to feel noticeably better. If you had any increased symptoms, make sure you review Meal Plan Troubleshooting 101 (see page 36).

In Week 2, we introduce nut milk or coconut milk, lactose-free dairy, and white and sweet potatoes. If you know you don't tolerate any of these items, simply switch out any recipes in the menu plan for another one marked Calming Menu+, Week 1+, or Week 2+.

WEEK 2 SHOPPING LIST

Canned and Bottled Items

- ☐ Capers, small jar (1)
- ☐ Crushed tomatoes or tomato sauce, organic, without garlic (2 cups)
- ☐ Olives, without garlic, for snacking

Dairy and Eggs

- ☐ Aged cheese (30 days or more), for snacking (3 ounces)
- ☐ Butter, organic grass-fed, or ghee (1 pound)
- ☐ Eggs, pastured (1 dozen large)
- ☐ Milk, lactose-free, nut, or coconut, without gums if possible, small bottle (1), optional
- ☐ Parmesan cheese, aged 30 days or more (8 ounces)

- ☐ Yogurt, 1 of the following:
  - 1 jar of premade 24-hour yogurt (White Mountain Bulgarian brand)
  - 1 batch of 24-Hour Yogurt (page 84)

Meat and Poultry

- ☐ Bacon (1 pound)
- ☐ Beef, grass-fed chuck or rump roast, 1 (3 pounds)
- ☐ Beef or turkey, ground, grass-fed (2 pounds)
- ☐ Chicken, organic legs (2 pounds) and organic livers (1 pound)
- ☐ Deli meat, roast turkey or roast beef, without garlic or other high-FODMAP additives (6 slices)
- ☐ Lamb chops, grass-fed organic (8 baby chops)
- ☐ Pork, ground (2 pounds)

Seafood

- ☐ Mahi-mahi, fillets (4)
- ☐ Salmon, 5-ounce fillets (2)

Pantry Items

- ☐ Avocado oil
- ☐ Broth, 1 of the following:
  - 1 batch of Low-FODMAP Vegetable Broth (page 90)
  - 4 cups of low-FODMAP chicken or vegetable broth (see Resources, page 206)
  - 2 batches of Pressure Cooker Bone Broth (page 92)
- ☐ Clover honey, pasteurized
- ☐ Coconut oil
- ☐ Collagen hydrolysate or collagen peptides (Great Lakes or Vital Proteins brand)
- ☐ Extra-virgin olive oil
- ☐ Garlic oil
- ☐ Maple syrup
- ☐ MCT oil
- ☐ Nut butter, low-FODMAP
- ☐ Pumpkin pie spice
- ☐ White rice
- ☐ White rice noodles, made with white rice or white rice flour and water only, 8-ounce package (1)
- ☐ Yellow curry powder

Produce

- ☐ Avocados (2 small)
- ☐ Banana (1)
- ☐ Bell pepper, organic red (1 medium)
- ☐ Blueberries, fresh or frozen (1 cup)
- ☐ Bok choy (1 large, or 3 or 4 baby)
- ☐ Carrots (2 pounds; prewashed, peeled baby carrots are easiest)
- ☐ Celery, organic (1 bunch)
- ☐ Chives, fresh (1 bunch)
- ☐ Cilantro, fresh (2 bunches)
- ☐ Dill, fresh (1 bunch)
- ☐ Ginger, fresh (5-inch piece)
- ☐ Green beans (1½ pounds)
- ☐ Lemon (1)
- ☐ Limes (2)
- ☐ Microgreens, small package (1)
- ☐ Orange, organic (1)
- ☐ Parsley, fresh (1 bunch)
- ☐ Potatoes, organic red (2 pounds)
- ☐ Rosemary, fresh (1 bunch)
- ☐ Sage, fresh (1 bunch)
- ☐ Scallions (1 bunch)
- ☐ Spinach, fresh, prewashed organic, 10-ounce bag (1)
- ☐ Strawberries, fresh or frozen organic (4 cups)
- ☐ Sweet potatoes (4 medium)
- ☐ Swiss chard (2 bunches)
- ☐ Tomatoes, organic (3 small)
- ☐ Zucchini (4 small)

Week 2 Meal Prep

- Make or purchase 24-Hour Yogurt (page 84)
- Make Pressure Cooker Bone Broth (page 92) or purchase low-FODMAP bone broth (see Resources, page 206).
- Double the recipe for Maple-Sage Breakfast Sausage (page 81) and divide in half. Make half into patties as instructed in the recipe, cook, and use for Week 2. Freeze the other half to use in the Sausage and Sweet Potato Hash (page 82) on Saturday.
- Make Creamy Cardamom Custard (page 183), Detoxifying Vegetable Soup (page 91), and Sweet Potato Chili (page 97).
- Make Deli Meat Roll-Ups (page 134) for Monday lunch.

EASY WEEKDAY COOKING

- Weeknight dinners are made nightly and are designed to be quick and simple.
- Make Cinnamon Rice (page 79) on Monday night. If desired, you can also make the bacon in advance.

- Double or halve recipes depending on leftovers used later in the week and if you're eating with other people.
- If the amount of cooking is stressful for you, pick some recipes from Week 1 that you found easy to make and swap them in for those recipes in Week 2 that you think may take more time than you have. Remember, you want a combination of healthy fats, carbohydrates, and protein in each meal.
- Take extra snacks with you if you think you may have a longer day at work. Because you're on a special diet, it's reassuring to have food with you so you don't have to resort to eating something off your diet in unexpected circumstances.
- If you need to switch out a recipe because you don't like or tolerate one listed, choose one denoted by Calming Menu+, Week 1+ or Week 2+, meaning it is appropriate for the Calming Menu, Week 1, or Week 2.
- Water isn't noted on the diet—stay hydrated; it affects your digestion.
- Eat the amount that is right for you. Calorie intake will vary by person.
- All the recipes are designed to be low FODMAP in one serving. If you are going to eat more than one serving at a meal, check to make sure the ingredients are low FODMAP in the amount you're eating, particularly for recipes that include sweet potatoes or green beans.

Week 2 Menu

	Monday	Tuesday	Wednesday	
BREAKFAST	24-Hour Yogurt with Strawberry Compote (page 84) Maple-Sage Breakfast Sausage (page 81)	Detoxifying Vegetable Soup (page 91) Cinnamon Rice (page 79) 2 or 3 bacon slices	Maple-Sage Breakfast Sausage (page 81) Creamy Cardamom Custard (page 183) Sautéed Spinach (page 107)	
LUNCH	Detoxifying Vegetable Soup (page 91) Deli Meat Roll-Ups (page 134)	Sweet Potato Chili (page 97)	Detoxifying Vegetable Soup (page 91) Garlic-Parmesan Chicken Legs (page 137)	
DINNER	Sweet Potato Chili (page 97) Sautéed Spinach (page 107)	Garlic-Parmesan Chicken Legs (page 137) Tender Swiss Chard (page 113)	Honey-Mustard Salmon (page 162) Dilly Potato Salad (page 123)	
DESSERTS OR SNACKS	Pressure Cooker Bone Broth (page 92)	Sautéed Banana (page 171)	Olives and aged cheese	

	Thursday	Friday	Saturday	Sunday
	Detoxifying Vegetable Soup (page 91) Savory Egg Scramble (page 78) Cinnamon Rice (page 79)	Satisfying Smoothie (page 175)	24-Hour Yogurt with Strawberry Compote (page 84) Sausage and Sweet Potato Hash (page 82)	Detoxifying Vegetable Soup (page 91) Creamy Cardamom Custard (page 183)
	Sweet Potato Chili (page 97)	Detoxifying Vegetable Soup (page 91) Slow Cooker Roast Beef (page 144)	Rosemary Lamb Chops (page 147) Buttery Rice Noodles (page 122)	Bacon-Wrapped Chicken Livers with Ranch Dressing (page 138) Carrot-Ginger Purée (page 106)
	Slow Cooker Roast Beef (page 144) Tender Swiss Chard (page 113)	Rosemary Lamb Chops (page 147) Sautéed Spinach (page 107) Dilly Potato Salad (page 123)	Bacon-Wrapped Chicken Livers with Ranch Dressing (page 138) Balsamic Green Beans (page 111)	Mahi-Mahi with Avocado-Lime Butter (page 163) Carrot-Ginger Purée (page 106)
	Pressure Cooker Bone Broth (page 92)	Creamy Cardamom Custard (page 183)	Pressure Cooker Bone Broth (page 92)	Olives and aged cheese

WEEK 3

You're halfway through the month! Hopefully you are feeling healthy and you're also able to connect symptoms with certain foods by keeping your food diary up to date. Remember, you can stay in Week 2 or even go back to the Calming Menu as needed. As new foods are introduced, you may encounter symptoms, which is your body's way of providing information. If you are unsure of your tolerance for a new food, reduce or remove it for now.

In Week 3, raw fruits and vegetables, zucchini, and dark chocolate are introduced (yes, chocolate!). If you're not sure of your tolerance for raw fruit or vegetables, start with very small portions and work up to a side salad. If you know you don't tolerate a specific item, simply switch out any recipes in the menu plan for another one marked Calming Menu+, Week 1+, Week 2+, or Week 3+.

WEEK 3 SHOPPING LIST

Canned and Bottled Items

- ☐ Anchovy paste, wild-caught, small tube (1)
- ☐ Fish sauce, gluten-free (preferably Red Boat brand), small bottle (1)

Dairy and Eggs

- ☐ Butter, organic grass-fed, or ghee (1 pound)
- ☐ Cheddar cheese, aged 30 days or more, shredded (1 cup)
- ☐ Coconut milk, full-fat, or lactose-free half-and-half (1½ cups)
- ☐ Eggs, pastured (2 dozen large)
- ☐ Milk, lactose-free, nut, or coconut, small container (1), optional
- ☐ Parmesan cheese, aged 30 days or more, grated (⅔ cup)

- ☐ Yogurt, 1 of the following:
  - 1 jar of premade 24-hour yogurt (White Mountain Bulgarian brand)
  - 1 batch of 24-Hour Yogurt (page 84)

Meat and Poultry

- ☐ Bacon (1 pound)
- ☐ Beef, grass-fed chuck or rump roast, 1 (2 to 3 pounds)
- ☐ Beef, ground, grass-fed (1 pound)
- ☐ Chicken, rotisserie (seasoned with salt and pepper only) or whole organic, 1 (2 to 3 pounds)
- ☐ Deli meat, organic (6 slices)
- ☐ Pork, ground (4 pounds)

Seafood

- ☐ Salmon, wild-caught, or other wild-caught fish (1 pound)
- ☐ Shrimp, raw (1 pound)

Pantry Items

- [ ] Broth, 1 of the following:
  - 1 batch of Low-FODMAP Vegetable Broth (page 90)
  - 8 to 12 cups of low-FODMAP chicken or beef broth (see Resources, page 206)
  - 2 batches of Pressure Cooker Bone Broth (page 92)
- [ ] Chinese five-spice powder
- [ ] Chocolate, dark (6 ounces)
- [ ] Clover honey, pasteurized
- [ ] Coconut, shredded unsweetened, small bag (1) (Let's Do … Organic brand recommended)
- [ ] Coconut butter or manna, small jar (1)
- [ ] Coconut oil
- [ ] Coconut water
- [ ] Corn tortillas, optional
- [ ] Garlic oil
- [ ] Kalamata or Picholine olives, pitted (⅓ cup)
- [ ] Maple syrup
- [ ] Nut butter, low-FODMAP
- [ ] Rice wine vinegar
- [ ] White rice
- [ ] White rice noodles, made with white rice or white rice flour and water only, 8-ounce package (1)

Produce

- [ ] Arugula, prewashed, 6-ounce bag (1)
- [ ] Avocados (4)
- [ ] Baby greens or butter lettuce, prewashed (1 bag)
- [ ] Basil, fresh (1 bunch)
- [ ] Bell peppers, organic green (1 small) and organic red (3 medium)
- [ ] Blueberries, organic (2 pints)
- [ ] Butter lettuce (1 large head or 2 small heads)
- [ ] Carrots, shredded (1 pound) and regular or baby carrots (3 pounds)
- [ ] Celery, organic (1 bunch)
- [ ] Cherry tomatoes, organic (2 pints)
- [ ] Chives, fresh (2 bunches)
- [ ] Cilantro, fresh (3 bunches)
- [ ] Cucumber (1)
- [ ] English cucumber (1)
- [ ] Ginger, fresh (4-inch piece)
- [ ] Grapes, organic (1 bunch)
- [ ] Green beans (½ pound)
- [ ] Lemons (7)
- [ ] Limes (5)
- [ ] Mint, fresh (1 bunch)
- [ ] Oranges, organic (7 large)
- [ ] Parsley, fresh (2 bunches)
- [ ] Potatoes, organic white russet (2 pounds)
- [ ] Raspberries, organic (1 pint)
- [ ] Rhubarb (8 stalks)
- [ ] Romaine lettuce (1 head)
- [ ] Sage, fresh (1 bunch)
- [ ] Scallions (2 bunches)
- [ ] Spinach, fresh, prewashed organic, 10-ounce bag (1)
- [ ] Strawberries, fresh organic (1 pint) and fresh or frozen organic (4 cups)
- [ ] Sweet potatoes (2 large and 2 small)
- [ ] Thai basil, fresh (1 bunch)
- [ ] Tomatoes, organic (9 large and 1 small)
- [ ] Zucchini (8 medium or 10 small)

Other

- [ ] Vermouth, dry (1 cup)
- [ ] Whiskey, optional (3 tablespoons)

Week 3 Meal Prep

WEEKEND BULK COOKING

- Purchase rotisserie chicken (seasoned with salt and pepper only) or roast a whole organic chicken.
- Make Pressure Cooker Bone Broth (page 92) or purchase low-FODMAP bone broth (see Resources, page 206).
- Leftover 24-Hour Yogurt (page 84) from last week will be used for one breakfast. If you've already used it up, make or purchase more.
- Prepare Beef Burrito Bowls (page 154) for lunch; refrigerate and/or freeze.
- Make Breakfast Egg Muffins (page 80) and freeze some for later.
- Make Fruit Salad with Mint-Lime Dressing (page 101).
- Make Strawberry Compote (page 83).
- Make Detoxifying Vegetable Soup (page 91).

EASY WEEKDAY COOKING

- Weeknight dinners are made nightly and are designed to be quick and simple.
- Homemade Electrolyte Drink (page 177) can be put together over the weekend or on Tuesday night.
- Make Caesar Salad Dressing (page 197) on Monday night for Tuesday lunch.
- Snacks and desserts can be made over the weekend or the evening before it's on the menu.

- Double or halve recipes depending on leftovers used later in the week and if you're eating with other people.
- This week's menu is full of fresh and cooked vegetables. If it is too much for you, remove some vegetable-heavy dishes and bring back some simple soup or meat recipes from the previous weeks.
- Note that when symptoms appear you can sometimes have a particular food with less frequency rather than cutting it out altogether.
- Eat the amount that is right for you. Calorie intake will vary by person.
- Hardboiled eggs are an easily portable breakfast or snack and can be purchased precooked.
- Buy precut vegetables to save time as needed.
- If you need to switch out a recipe because you don't like or tolerate one listed, choose one denoted by anything other than Week 4+.
- Water isn't noted on the diet—stay hydrated; it affects your digestion.
- All the recipes are designed to be low FODMAP in one serving. If you are going to eat more than one serving at a meal, check to make sure the ingredients are low FODMAP in the amount you're eating, particularly for recipes that include sweet potatoes or green beans.

Week 3 Menu

	Monday	Tuesday	Wednesday	
BREAKFAST	Breakfast Egg Muffins (page 80) Cinnamon Sweet Potatoes (page 85)	24-Hour Yogurt with Strawberry Compote (page 84) Maple-Sage Breakfast Sausage (page 81)	Homemade Electrolyte Drink (page 177) Breakfast Egg Muffins (page 80) Cinnamon Rice (page 79)	
LUNCH	Detoxifying Vegetable Soup (page 91) Beef Burrito Bowls (page 154)	Detoxifying Vegetable Soup (page 91) Chicken Caesar Salad (page 102)	Chilled Tomato Soup (page 98) Beef Burrito Bowls (page 154)	
DINNER	Orange and Olive Salad (page 99) Simple Roast Chicken (page 132) Creamy Mashed Potatoes (page 124)	Chilled Tomato Soup (page 98) Fish Tacos (page 167)	Saucy Vegetable Rice Noodle Bowl (page 126) with leftover Simple Roast Chicken	
DESSERTS OR SNACKS	Pressure Cooker Bone Broth (page 92)	Vanilla-Orange Fat Bombs (page 184)	Detoxifying Vegetable Soup (page 91)	

	Thursday	Friday	Saturday	Sunday
	Maple-Sage Breakfast Sausage (page 81) Cinnamon Sweet Potatoes (page 85)	Satisfying Smoothie (page 175)	Blueberry-Coconut Milk (page 176) Savory Egg Scramble (page 78)	Sausage and Sweet Potato Hash (page 82) Fried eggs
	Saucy Vegetable Rice Noodle Bowl (page 126) with leftover Simple Roast Chicken	Pressure Cooker Bone Broth (page 92) Asian Ground Pork in Lettuce Cups (page 155)	Detoxifying Vegetable Soup (page 91) Deli Meat Roll-Ups (page 134)	Tomato-Garlic Shrimp (page 161) Carrot-Ginger Purée (page 106)
	Fruit Salad with Mint-Lime Dressing (page 101) Asian Ground Pork in Lettuce Cups (page 155)	Pesto Zoodles with Chicken (page 139)	Tomato-Garlic Shrimp (page 161) Carrot-Ginger Purée (page 106)	Slow Cooker Roast Beef (page 144) Sautéed Spinach (page 107)
	Pressure Cooker Bone Broth (page 92)	Roasted Orange Rhubarb (page 185)	Zucchini Chips (page 114)	Chocolate Pots de Crème (page 188)

WEEK 4

This is the homestretch! After three weeks of being on the meal plan, you should be acquiring a far greater understanding of your symptoms and what you tolerate, as well as how frequently you can eat certain items. Some people will have experienced desired weight loss over this period from eating less-processed food and fewer carbo-hydrates. For those who have been experiencing unwanted weight loss, remember to review the Meal Plan Troubleshooting 101 section (page 36).

Also, if you've begun to have more symptoms that are unmanageable, stick with an earlier menu until you come to a neutral point with manageable symptoms. Or you can introduce some items from the Week 4 menu without adding everything in it. During Week 4, we introduce quinoa and nuts. You should be very proud for taking these steps to learn more about yourself. Here's to your health!

WEEK 4 SHOPPING LIST

Canned and Bottled Items

- ☐ Chopped tomatoes, organic, 14-ounce can (1)
- ☐ Tomato paste, organic, 14-ounce can (1)

Dairy and Eggs

- ☐ Butter, organic grass-fed, or ghee (1 pound)
- ☐ Eggs, pastured (1 dozen large)
- ☐ Milk, lactose-free, coconut, or nut, without gums if possible, small container (1), optional
- ☐ Yogurt, 1 of the following:
  - • 1 jar of premade 24-hour yogurt (White Mountain Bulgarian brand)
  - • 1 batch of 24-Hour Yogurt (page 84)

Meat and Poultry

- ☐ Bacon (1 pound)
- ☐ Beef, grass-fed boneless sirloin, rib eye, or similar steak (1½ pounds)
- ☐ Beef, grass-fed chuck or rump roast, 1 (2 pounds)
- ☐ Beef, short ribs (5 pounds)
- ☐ Chicken, rotisserie (seasoned with salt and pepper only) or whole organic, 1 (2 to 3 pounds)
- ☐ Chicken, skinless thighs (1½ pounds)
- ☐ Pork, ground (2 pounds)

Seafood

- ☐ Cod, fillets (4)
- ☐ Swordfish, fillets (1½ pounds)

Pantry Items

- ☐ Arrowroot powder
- ☐ Bread, gluten-free country-style loaf (1)
- ☐ Broth, 1 of the following:
  - 1 batch of Low-FODMAP Vegetable Broth (page 90)
  - 8 to 12 cups of low-FODMAP chicken or beef broth (see Resources, page 206)
  - 2 batches of Pressure Cooker Bone Broth (page 92)
- ☐ Chocolate, dark, 70% cacao or higher (⅓ cup) and unsweetened (½ ounce)
- ☐ Clover honey, pasteurized
- ☐ Cornmeal, gluten-free
- ☐ Corn tortillas, optional
- ☐ Flour, gluten-free
- ☐ Gelatin powder, grass-fed (such as Great Lakes brand)
- ☐ Maple syrup
- ☐ Nuts, mixed, including almonds, macadamias, walnuts, and pecans (4 cups), and pecans (1 pound)
- ☐ Peppermint extract
- ☐ Quinoa
- ☐ White rice
- ☐ White rice noodles, made with white rice or white rice flour and water only, 8-ounce package (1)
- ☐ White wine vinegar
- ☐ Whole cane sugar (such as Sucanat)

Produce

- ☐ Avocado (1)
- ☐ Basil, fresh (2 bunches)
- ☐ Bell peppers, organic red (3)
- ☐ Blueberries (1 pint)
- ☐ Broccoli (3 heads)
- ☐ Butter or romaine lettuce leaves, optional
- ☐ Carrots, shredded (24 ounces) and whole (1)
- ☐ Celery, organic (1 bunch)
- ☐ Cherry tomatoes, organic (2 pints)
- ☐ Chives, fresh (1 bunch)
- ☐ Cilantro, fresh (2 bunches)
- ☐ Ginger, fresh (7-inch piece)
- ☐ Green beans (1 pound)
- ☐ Kale (2 bunches)
- ☐ Lemons (2)
- ☐ Limes (6)
- ☐ Oranges, organic (2)
- ☐ Parsley, fresh (1 bunch)
- ☐ Potatoes, organic white russet (2 pounds)
- ☐ Sage, fresh (1 bunch)
- ☐ Scallions (2 bunches)
- ☐ Spinach, fresh, prewashed organic, 10-ounce bags (2)
- ☐ Strawberries, fresh or frozen organic (4 cups)
- ☐ Sweet potatoes (2 medium)
- ☐ Swiss chard (2 bunches)
- ☐ Thyme, fresh
- ☐ Zucchini (2 small or 1 medium)

Other

- ☐ Red wine, dry
- ☐ Sherry, dry (1 cup)

Week 4 Meal Prep

- Purchase rotisserie chicken (seasoned with salt and pepper only) or roast a whole chicken.
- Make Pressure Cooker Bone Broth (page 92) or purchase low-FODMAP bone broth (see Resources, page 206).
- Make or purchase 24-Hour Yogurt (page 84).
- Make Breakfast Egg Muffins (page 80) or unfreeze some you made previously.
- Make Detoxifying Vegetable Soup (page 91).
- Make Saucy Vegetable Rice Noodle Bowl (page 126) for lunch to go.
- Make Corn Bread (page 86).

EASY WEEKDAY COOKING

- Weeknight dinners are made nightly and are designed to be quick and simple.
- Snacks and desserts can be made over the weekend or the evening before it's on the menu.
- Start Slow Cooker Beef Tacos (page 152) on Wednesday night and refrigerate on Thursday morning, or start on Thursday morning for dinner Thursday night.

- Double or halve recipes depending on leftovers used later in the week and if you're eating with other people.
- If you don't react well to whole nuts, go back to having nut butter as a snack.
- Note that when symptoms appear, sometimes you can have something with less frequency rather than cutting it out altogether.
- Eat the amount that is right for you. Calorie intake will vary by person.
- Hardboiled eggs are an easily portable breakfast or snack and can be purchased precooked.
- Buy precut vegetables to save time as needed.
- If you need to switch out a recipe because you don't like or tolerate one listed, choose one that you like and tolerate.
- Water isn't noted on the diet—stay hydrated; it affects your digestion.
- All the recipes are designed to be low FODMAP in one serving. If you are going to eat more than one serving at a meal, check to make sure the ingredients are low FODMAP in the amount you're eating, particularly for recipes that include sweet potatoes or green beans.

Week 4 Menu

	Monday	Tuesday	Wednesday	
BREAKFAST	Detoxifying Vegetable Soup (page 91) 2 bacon slices Corn Bread (page 86)	Pressure Cooker Bone Broth (page 92) Savory Egg Scramble (page 78) Cinnamon Rice (page 79)	Maple-Sage Breakfast Sausage (page 81) Sautéed Spinach (page 107) Corn Bread (page 86)	
LUNCH	Saucy Vegetable Rice Noodle Bowl (page 126)	Saucy Vegetable Rice Noodle Bowl (page 126) with leftover Simple Steak	Pressure Cooker General Tso's Chicken (page 140) Basic White Rice (page 120) Sautéed Spinach (page 107)	
DINNER	Simple Steak (page 145) Broccoli with Lemon-Mustard Butter (page 116)	Pressure Cooker General Tso's Chicken (page 140) Basic White Rice (page 120) Sautéed Spinach (page 107)	Curry Quinoa Stir-Fry (page 128)	
DESSERTS OR SNACKS	Mixed Nuts (page 178)	Kale Chips (page 115)	Detoxifying Vegetable Soup (page 91)	

Thursday	Friday	Saturday	Sunday
Pressure Cooker Bone Broth (page 92) Breakfast Egg Muffins (page 80) Cinnamon Rice (page 79)	Detoxifying Vegetable Soup (page 91) Maple-Sage Breakfast Sausage (page 81) Corn Bread (page 86)	Satisfying Smoothie (page 175) Breakfast Egg Muffins (page 80)	24-Hour Yogurt with Strawberry Compote (page 84) 2 bacon slices
Curry Quinoa Stir-Fry (page 128)	Slow Cooker Beef Tacos (page 152)	Cod with Tomato-Basil Sauce (page 166) Tender Swiss Chard (page 113)	Spanish Short Ribs (page 156) Creamy Mashed Potatoes (page 124) Honey-Mustard Green Beans (page 108)
Slow Cooker Beef Tacos (page 152)	Cod with Tomato-Basil Sauce (page 166) Tender Swiss Chard (page 113)	Spanish Short Ribs (page 156) Creamy Mashed Potatoes (page 124) Honey-Mustard Green Beans (page 108)	Ginger-Lime Swordfish Skewers (page 165) Sweet Potato Wedges (page 125)
Peppermint Marshmallows (page 189)	Pressure Cooker Bone Broth (page 92)	Chocolate-Pecan Nut Butter (page 191)	Pressure Cooker Bone Broth (page 92)

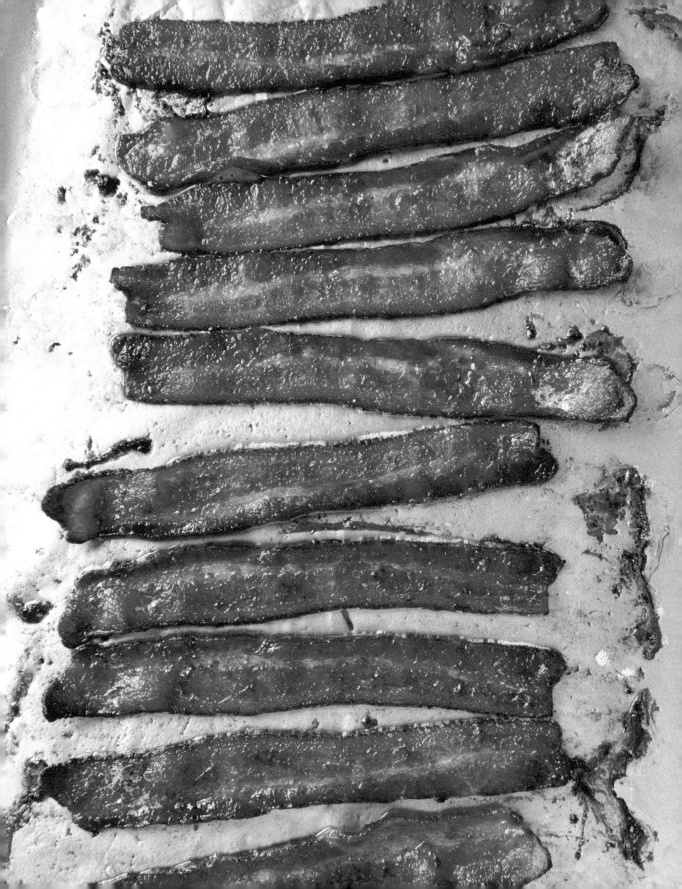

Beyond the 4 Weeks

Congratulations on your healing journey.

You've started a new diet and adopted a new way of thinking. You've learned shortcuts, reimagined meal times, and supported yourself with four weeks of healthy, healing foods. Long-term healing from SIBO is often not a linear path. It requires us to stick to helpful habits and continue to seek answers to lingering issues. Some people may begin to heal from this four-week meal plan, while for others it will be a longer and more involved journey. Wherever you are on your path, this chapter supports you with tips on testing new low- and high-FODMAP foods as well as ideas for assembling quick and nutritious meals. Since having SIBO can be isolating, and connecting to family and friends is key, we also review ways to enjoy eating out, going on vacation, and attending events. Continue to look for ways to feel whole as you heal.

TESTING NEW FOODS

After the monthlong diet, begin to add more foods to your meals that you're currently not eating but that are low-FODMAP. There's not a one-size-fits-all option when it comes to food testing. Match the food introduction style to your current sensitivity level:

1. **Highly Sensitive.** Eat a small amount of the new item, such as 1 teaspoon of 24-Hour Yogurt (page 84) or 2 tablespoons of white rice, and wait 48 hours to assess symptoms. If you react negatively, wait three to four weeks before retesting the food. If you don't react, add the new item to your diet. Eat it a couple of times a week at first and then try it more frequently.

2. **Moderately Sensitive.** Eat small amounts of an item (one-third of a regular portion size). The next day, eat a larger amount (two-thirds of a portion size), and on the final day, eat a full portion. This tests the amount and frequency at which you tolerate an item.

3. **Low Sensitivity.** Eat a small amount of an item three times in one day, or eat a progressively larger amount of the same item in the same day. In this mode, you test both frequency and amounts. Back off on the frequency and then the amount as needed.

If you have a reaction, get back to a neutral point before trying another food. Don't add new foods in the midst of a flare. Instead, go back to eating simple foods for a couple of days, take the supplements that support your digestion, and test a new food when you feel better.

TESTING HIGH-FODMAP FOODS

Not all people react to each FODMAP type. After a negative SIBO test, it is helpful to stay on a low-FODMAP diet for at least a month and then test and add specific FODMAPs back into your diet.

It is easiest to test foods with one high FODMAP at first to ascertain which FODMAP may be triggering a reaction. Test any of the following foods that have only one high FODMAP:

- **Fructose.** asparagus OR mango OR canned artichoke hearts

- **Lactose.** plain yogurt OR milk OR ice cream

- **Sorbitol.** avocado OR green beans

- Mannitol. mushrooms OR cauliflower OR sweet potato

- GOS. green or red boiled lentils OR cashews

- FOS (oligo-fructans). leek OR garlic clove

HOLIDAYS, BIRTHDAYS, AND SOCIAL EVENTS

Use these simple strategies to manage eating away from home. While managing your physical health, it's important to take care of your emotional health as well, and being connected to friends and family is an important part of that.

Eat before you go. If you're going to a work event or social party where you're unfamiliar with the host, it may be less stressful to eat ahead of time. You won't feel pressure to eat a full meal at the event but can pick and choose what works for you.

Bring food with you. If you're attending a cocktail party, take your own appetizer. Pour yourself some water with a lime wedge if you aren't up for an alcoholic drink. For a dinner party, discuss the menu with the host beforehand, if you feel comfortable. As needed, ask if it's okay to bring all or part of your own meal.

Choose wisely. Avoid dips and casseroles with unknown ingredients. Nibble on olives, one or two raw vegetables, or nuts to have something on your plate.

Boundaries. If someone questions what you're eating, remember, you get to choose how much to disclose or whether to talk about it at all. It's fine to talk about your health situation if you want to share, but it's also fine to change the subject or simply tell someone you don't want to discuss it with them. It's also an option to turn down an invitation. Remember to take care of yourself and see what feels right in each situation.

RESTAURANTS

Restaurants are about hospitality. If you know where you'll be eating, look up the menu online or call ahead and speak with the chef. Call in the early afternoon so someone will be there but not in the heat of getting ready for service. Most chefs, especially at nicer establishments, will be helpful if you are very clear about when you're coming in and your specific needs. It tends to be easiest to order a protein and specific (well-cooked) vegetables without sauce, seasoned with just salt and pepper, and with a specific oil or fat as needed. If you are able to eat a side salad, most restaurants can also do a simple salad with lemon juice or vinegar and olive oil.

If you aren't able to call ahead, that's okay. Many restaurants are fully aware of special dietary considerations and food allergies—just be very specific when speaking with your waiter. If the waitperson doesn't seem to understand, it might be helpful to add that you have an allergy or need to make sure your order is accurate so you don't get sick.

VACATION

Vacation is a time for relaxation and rejuvenation—not a time to stress about your diet. Keep these tips in mind and take full advantage of your time away.

Stay. Rent all or part of a house with kitchen access to ensure you have cooking and storing options. If you choose a hotel, ask for a room with a mini refrigerator so you can store snacks or breakfast items.

Snack. Pack your own meal when flying, and bring enough snacks for your entire stay. As needed, you can typically buy olives, nuts, nut butter, lactose-free yogurt, rice cakes, or tortilla chips, depending on what you tolerate, at your location.

Shop. Check out your destination in advance to see what grocery stores are available. Choose deli items that list all the ingredients.

Don't stress. Once you've done as much planning and prep as possible, do your best to let go. People tend to be able to eat a wider variety of foods while on vacation—probably because they're feeling less stressed. So if you decide to try a new food or eat outside your diet, breathe deeply and enjoy yourself.

Meals on the Go

Nobody says you have to cook every night of the week! It's easy to build a quick meal with what is already in your refrigerator. Do a quick review of your food options, warm up components as needed, grab a bowl, and start assembling.

Grains or starches. Use grains or starches as a base if you tolerate them. Try white rice, quinoa, mashed potato, or up to ½ cup of sweet potato.

Veggies. Pick one or two leftover or fresh vegetables to create the next layer. Try sautéed spinach or arugula, carrots, green beans, soft lettuces, bell peppers, tomatoes, zucchini, or cucumber.

Protein. Add your favorite protein, whether that's leftover chicken, fish, or steak, hardboiled egg slices, or a freshly poached egg.

Sauce or dressing. Sauces can be used over the first three layers or they can be mixed in with an individual layer. For instance, sauté quinoa with curry powder, coconut oil, and coconut milk as a base layer that also creates a sauce. Or add a cold dressing or warm sauce, such as a chimichurri, hollandaise, or vinaigrette.

Toppings. Let your imagination run wild! Toppings may include herbs, cheese, nuts, or a slice of avocado.

POSSIBLE COMBINATIONS:

- Cold rice + salmon + cucumber + tomato + lemon vinaigrette + aged feta + dill
- Quinoa + chicken + sautéed bell peppers + coconut milk + curry powder + slivered almonds
- Sweet potato + sautéed spinach + flank steak + poached egg + hollandaise sauce + parsley

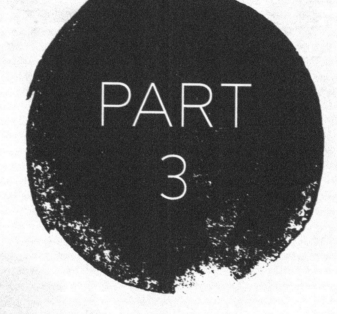

PART
3

The Recipes

Now for the fun part: the recipes! Granted, with everyone's different tolerances and specific tastes, not every recipe here will work for you. That's why the recipes are specifically marked with symbols for dietary considerations, including dairy-free, gluten-free, nut-free, vegan, and vegetarian. They also include helpful tips and information. As you try the different recipes and get used to noting your symptoms and tolerances, you'll be able to make the recipes your own by adding or substituting other ingredients or spices. These recipes are designed to be nutrient-dense, delicious, and, most important, easy and approachable. Enjoy!

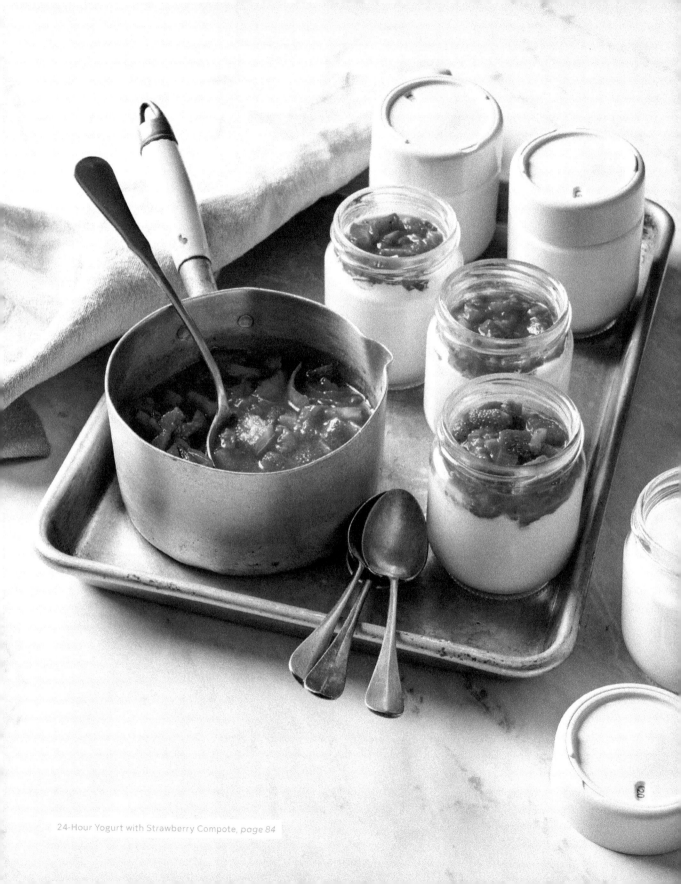

24-Hour Yogurt with Strawberry Compote, page 84

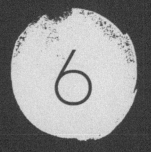

Breakfast

Savory Egg Scramble

This is a simple yet satisfying egg scramble that can be easily and quickly whipped up on a weekday.

Serves 2

PREP TIME: **10 minutes**

COOK TIME: **15 minutes**

2 tablespoons coconut oil, ghee, or organic grass-fed butter

1 small zucchini, peeled, cut lengthwise, and sliced into half-moons

1 cup fresh spinach, chopped

4 large eggs, beaten

Salt

Freshly ground black pepper

¼ cup chopped tomato (optional)

¼ avocado, chopped (optional)

2 tablespoons chopped fresh chives (optional; omit if on the Calming Menu)

1. Melt the coconut oil in a skillet over medium-high heat until sizzling but not smoking.

2. Add the zucchini. Cook for 5 to 10 minutes, or until very tender and beginning to brown.

3. Add the spinach. Cook for 1 minute.

4. Add the eggs and season with a generous sprinkle of salt and pepper. Cook, stirring, until the eggs reach your desired doneness. Divide the scrambled eggs between two plates.

5. Top with tomato, avocado, and chives (if using; recommended for Week 3 or after). Serve immediately.

Substitution tip: If you don't tolerate part of the egg, make this scramble using only egg yolks or only egg whites.

Per Serving (made with coconut oil and the optional items):
Calories: 302; Total Fat: 26g; Cholesterol: 372mg; Sodium: 156mg; Carbs: 4g; Sugar: 2g; Fiber: 1g; Protein: 14g

Cinnamon Rice

Cinnamon rice makes a delicious addition to breakfast. You can add milk (lactose-free, nut, or coconut) if you tolerate it to make the dish a little saucier.

Serves 1
PREP TIME: **5 minutes**
COOK TIME: **5 minutes**

1 cup cooked white rice

1 tablespoon organic grass-fed butter, ghee, or coconut oil

½ teaspoon ground cinnamon

¼ cup lactose-free, nut, or coconut milk (optional)

In a microwave-safe bowl or a small saucepan over medium-low heat, combine the rice, butter, cinnamon, and milk (if using). Microwave on high for 1 minute or cook, stirring occasionally, for 5 minutes, or until heated through. Serve warm.

Preparation tip: In Week 2, add a little sweetness by topping the rice with Strawberry Compote (page 83). In Week 3 or later, you can add some raw fruit, such as blueberries. If you prefer a vegan dish, use coconut oil and nut or coconut milk.

Per Serving (made with butter and lactose-free milk): Calories: 364; Total Fat: 20g; Cholesterol: 52mg; Sodium: 556mg; Carbs: 42g; Sugar: 3g; Fiber: 2g; Protein: 5g

Breakfast Egg Muffins

These egg muffins are so versatile that, depending on what you tolerate or prefer, you can pretty much substitute any type of cooked vegetables or meat you'd like.

Makes 12 muffins

PREP TIME: **10 minutes**

COOK TIME: **20 minutes**

1 tablespoon coconut oil, bacon fat, or ghee, melted (optional)

1 cup fresh spinach, chopped

4 cooked bacon slices, chopped

6 large eggs, beaten

¼ cup chopped fresh chives (optional; omit if on the Calming Menu)

1. Preheat the oven to 350°F. Line a 12-cup muffin tin with silicone molds or lightly oil the cups with the coconut oil.

2. In a medium bowl, combine the spinach, bacon, eggs, and chives (if using; recommended for Week 3 or after). Divide the mixture among the muffin cups. Bake for 15 to 20 minutes, or until the eggs set.

3. Serve immediately, or refrigerate or freeze.

Make-ahead tip: If your schedule is super busy, it's helpful to make large batches to freeze and thaw at the beginning of the week.

Per Serving (2 muffins, made with coconut oil): Calories: 179; Total Fat: 11g; Cholesterol: 190mg; Sodium: 18mg; Carbs: 9g; Sugar: 4g; Fiber: 5g; Protein: 15g

Maple-Sage Breakfast Sausage

Get the whole family involved in making this recipe. The kids can mix the sausage using their hands (clean ones!) and help shape the patties.

Serves 8

PREP TIME: **10 minutes**

COOK TIME: **20 minutes**

2 pounds ground pork

3 tablespoons finely chopped fresh sage leaves

2 tablespoons maple syrup

2 teaspoons sea salt

1 teaspoon pumpkin pie spice

1 teaspoon garlic oil

¼ teaspoon freshly ground black pepper

1 tablespoon avocado or coconut oil

1. In a medium bowl, combine the pork, sage, maple syrup, salt, pumpkin pie spice, garlic oil, and pepper. Mix thoroughly to combine. Form the mixture into 16 sausage patties.

2. Heat the avocado oil in a large skillet over medium-high heat.

3. When the oil is hot but not smoking, add the sausage patties, in batches if necessary, cooking them for 3 to 5 minutes per side. Leftovers can be refrigerated.

Make-ahead tip: This recipe can be doubled or tripled, and the cooked sausages can be stored in the freezer. Just pull out what you need for the week to save some prep time.

Per Serving (made with avocado oil): Calories: 335; Total Fat: 26g; Cholesterol: 82mg; Sodium: 645mg; Carbs: 4g; Sugar: 3g; Fiber: 0g; Protein: 19g

Sausage and Sweet Potato Hash

This simple hash can be topped with scrambled or fried eggs, or enjoyed all by itself.

Serves 4

PREP TIME: **10 minutes**

COOK TIME: **40 minutes**

2 cups cubed sweet potato
(about 2 small)

4 scallions, dark green parts
only, sliced and divided

½ teaspoon dried oregano

1 tablespoon garlic oil

2 tablespoons avocado oil, divided

1 organic red bell pepper, diced

1 pound Maple-Sage Breakfast
Sausage, uncooked (page 81)

1. Preheat the oven to 400°F.

2. On a baking sheet, combine the sweet potatoes, half the sliced scallions, the oregano, garlic oil, and 1 tablespoon of avocado oil. Mix to coat the sweet potatoes. Bake for 30 minutes, or until cooked through, stirring twice.

3. Meanwhile, heat the remaining tablespoon of avocado oil in a large skillet over medium-high heat.

4. Add the red bell pepper. Cook until soft.

5. Add the sausage. Cook for about 10 minutes, or until cooked through.

6. Add the sweet potato mixture and mix to combine thoroughly. Divide among four plates and serve immediately.

Ingredient tip: Stick to one serving of this hash for low FODMAP. White potatoes can also be substituted if you prefer.

Per Serving: Calories: 330; Total Fat: 24g; Cholesterol: 41mg; Sodium: 292mg; Carbs: 18g; Sugar: 7g; Fiber: 3g; Protein: 11g

Strawberry Compote

This compote can be made from fresh or frozen strawberries. It's great to have in the refrigerator to use as a topping for yogurt or pancakes, or just to enjoy by itself—warm or chilled.

Makes 4 cups

PREP TIME: **10 minutes**

COOK TIME: **20 minutes**

4 cups fresh or frozen organic strawberries

Zest of 1 organic orange

1 tablespoon freshly squeezed orange juice

2 tablespoons ghee, organic grass-fed butter, or coconut oil

1 tablespoon pasteurized clover honey (optional)

1. In a medium saucepan over medium heat, combine the strawberries, orange zest, orange juice, ghee, and honey (if using). Bring to a simmer. Reduce the heat to medium-low and cook for about 15 minutes, stirring frequently and breaking up the fruit into chunks with a wooden spoon, or until the mixture begins to thicken.

2. Keep refrigerated or frozen.

Ingredient tip: As strawberries are number-one on the Low-FODMAP Dirty Dozen list (see page 204), meaning they have the most pesticides of any fruit or vegetable when grown conventionally, it's important to buy them organic. In winter, look for frozen organic strawberries at Costco or other local supermarkets.

Per Serving (½ cup, made with ghee): Calories: 69; Total Fat: 4g; Cholesterol: 0mg; Sodium: 0mg; Carbs: 8g; Sugar: 6g; Fiber: 1g; Protein: 1g

24-Hour Yogurt with Strawberry Compote

This 24-hour yogurt has many beneficial probiotics and can be a helpful diet addition for people who are underweight. Additionally, it's just plain delicious and convenient.

Makes 8 cups of yogurt

PREP TIME: **5 minutes, plus 8 hours to chill**

COOK TIME: **24 hours**

2 quarts whole milk or half-and-half (or use the amount specified on your yogurt maker)

1 packet yogurt starter (such as Yogourmet)

Strawberry Compote (page 83) or pasteurized clover honey, for topping

1. Fill a shallow baking pan with ice and cold water and set aside.

2. In a saucepan over medium-high heat, heat the milk to 180°F, measured with an instant-read thermometer. Place the saucepan in the ice water until the milk cools to 110°F.

3. Place the yogurt starter in a large bowl.

4. Add ½ cup of milk from the saucepan to the yogurt starter and whisk well to combine.

5. Add the remaining milk to the starter. Whisk to combine.

6. Pour the mixture into a yogurt maker and heat at 110°F for 24 hours.

7. Refrigerate until firm, about 8 hours or overnight. Serve topped with the compote or clover honey.

SIBO tip: If you are sensitive and haven't tried yogurt before, start with a teaspoon or tablespoon and work your way up from there.

Per Serving (1 cup): Calories: 216; Total Fat: 12g; Cholesterol: 24mg; Sodium: 102mg; Carbs: 19g; Sugar: 19g; Fiber: 1g; Protein: 9g

Cinnamon Sweet Potatoes

One servisng of these sweet potatoes are low FODMAP and are an excellent source of vitamins A and C. These sweet potatoes are delicious for breakfast, and you can also make this dish savory rather than sweet simply by changing up the spice— try 1 teaspoon ground cumin or other spice you like instead of the cinnamon.

Serves 4

PREP TIME: **5 minutes**

2 cups mashed cooked
  sweet potato

1 teaspoon ground cinnamon

4 tablespoons ghee, organic
  grass-fed butter, or
  coconut oil, melted

In a medium bowl, combine the sweet potatoes, cinnamon, and ghee. Mash until creamy. Serve with toppings, as desired (see Ingredient tip).

Preparation tip: If you prefer a vegan dish, use coconut oil.

Ingredient tip: Sliced bananas, maple syrup, or nut butter make delicious toppings.

Per Serving (made with ghee): Calories: 194; Total Fat: 15g; Cholesterol: 0mg; Sodium: 37mg; Carbs: 14g; Sugar: 10g; Fiber: 5g; Protein: 2g

Corn Bread

This corn bread is ideal for breakfast or as an accompaniment to soup or an entrée.

Serves 9
PREP TIME: **10 minutes**
COOK TIME: **30 minutes**

6 tablespoons unsalted organic grass-fed butter, ghee, or coconut oil, melted, plus more for preparing the pan

1½ cups gluten-free flour, such as Bob's Red Mill all purpose baking flour

1½ cups gluten-free cornmeal

⅓ cup whole cane sugar, such as Sucanat (see Tip below)

2 teaspoons baking soda

2 teaspoons baking powder

1 teaspoon sea salt

2 large eggs

2 tablespoons pasteurized clover honey or maple syrup

1½ cups coconut milk, nut milk, or lactose-free milk

1. Preheat the oven to 400°F. Grease an 8-by-8-inch baking dish with butter and set aside.

2. In a large mixing bowl, combine the flour, cornmeal, cane sugar, baking soda, baking powder, and salt. Whisk until well mixed.

3. Make a well in the center of the mixture. Add the eggs and honey into the well and whisk them together.

4. Add the melted butter and whisk into the egg mixture.

5. Using a wooden spoon, mix the wet ingredients into the dry ingredients until just incorporated. Do not overmix. Pour the batter into the prepared pan and bake for 25 to 30 minutes, or until the top is light brown and a knife inserted into the center comes out clean.

6. Cut into 9 pieces and serve immediately, or let cool and keep refrigerated. Individual pieces can also be wrapped and frozen.

Ingredient tip: Sucanat is the least processed form of sugar and has an almost brown sugar taste and color. You can substitute granulated sugar for the Sucanat if you prefer.

Per Serving: Calories: 291; Total Fat: 12g; Cholesterol: 62mg; Sodium: 507mg; Carbs: 43g; Sugar: 12g; Fiber: 2g; Protein: 5g

Crème Brûlée French Toast

This is a fairly sweet and very special treat. It's really easy to put together the night before, and it makes an excellent brunch for company.

Serves 6

PREP TIME: **15 minutes, plus overnight to chill**

COOK TIME: **40 minutes**

8 tablespoons (1 stick) unsalted organic grass-fed butter or ghee

½ cup packed brown sugar

⅓ cup maple syrup

1 loaf, thick-cut country-style gluten-free bread

5 large eggs

1½ cups lactose-free half-and-half or full-fat coconut milk

1 teaspoon vanilla extract

¼ teaspoon sea salt

1. In a small saucepan over medium heat, combine the butter, brown sugar, and maple syrup. Cook, stirring, until melted and smooth. Pour the mixture into the bottom of a 9-by-13-inch baking dish.

2. Cut about 6 (1-inch) slices of the bread from the center portion of the loaf and arrange them in a single layer on top of the syrup mixture, squeezing them together to fit tightly.

3. In a medium bowl, whisk the eggs, half-and-half, vanilla, and salt until well combined. Pour the mixture evenly over the bread to coat. Cover and refrigerate overnight.

4. Remove the French toast from the refrigerator and preheat the oven to 350°F.

5. Uncover the French toast and bake for 35 to 40 minutes, or until light golden brown.

6. Cut into 6 pieces. Flip each piece over to serve. Top with fruit if you'd like (see Tip below) and serve immediately.

Preparation tip: To make this French toast extra tasty and beautiful, top with fresh berries or Sautéed Banana (page 171).

Per Serving: Calories: 707; Total Fat: 17g; Cholesterol: 180mg; Sodium: 409mg; Carbs: 119g; Sugar: 31g; Fiber: 10g; Protein: 26g

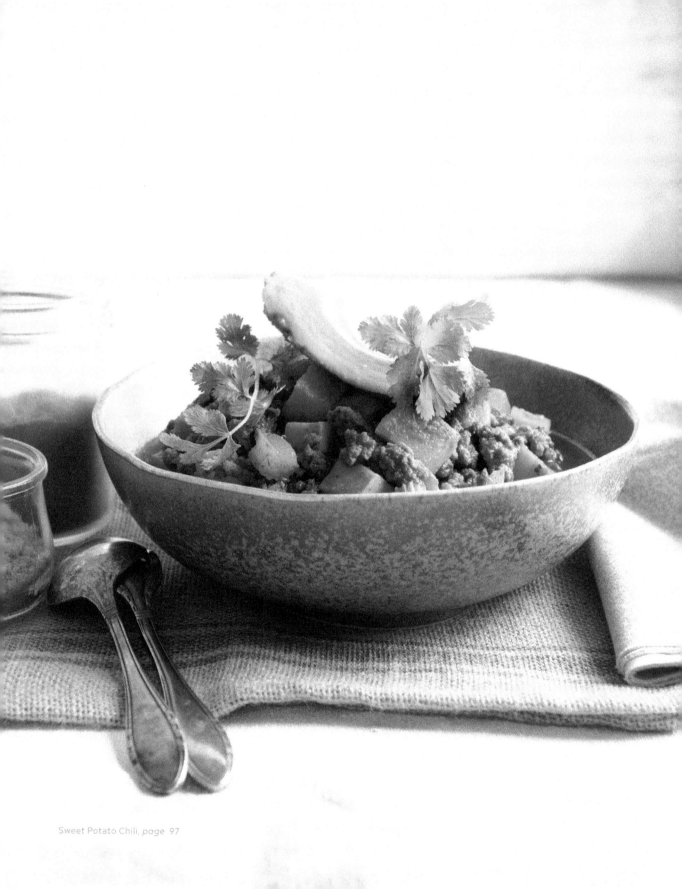

Sweet Potato Chili, *page 97*

Soups and Salads

7

Low-FODMAP Vegetable Broth

Throughout the week, save and freeze any leftover vegetable peels, scraps, or ends to use in this vegetable broth. If you don't have the time or inclination to make your own, see the Resources section (page 206) for online sources to purchase a low-FODMAP broth.

Makes 8 cups
PREP TIME: **20 minutes**
COOK TIME: **3 hours**

1 tablespoon coconut oil or ghee

½ cup to 2 cups vegetable scraps, like zucchini peels, carrot ends, or kale or Swiss chard ribs

3 carrots, chopped

4 celery stalks, chopped

4 scallions, dark green parts only, coarsely chopped

3 fresh rosemary sprigs

3 fresh thyme sprigs

½ cup fresh parsley leaves, roughly chopped

1 teaspoon peppercorns

3 quarts water

3 bay leaves

2 teaspoons sea salt, or to taste

1. Melt the coconut oil in a large stockpot over medium-high heat.

2. Add the vegetable scraps, carrots, celery, and scallions. Sauté the vegetables, stirring frequently, for about 5 minutes, or until softened and beginning to brown.

3. Add the rosemary, thyme, parsley, and peppercorns. Sauté for 3 minutes more.

4. Add the water, bay leaves, and salt. Bring the broth to a boil. Reduce the heat to low and simmer uncovered for 3 hours.

5. Strain the broth through a fine-mesh strainer and add more water as needed to make 8 cups total. Discard the solids. Keep the broth refrigerated for use within 3 to 4 days, or freeze (see Tip below).

Make-ahead tip: Make large batches of this broth and keep it in the freezer so you'll have it on hand to use as a soup base or in other recipes. Freeze the broth in ice cube trays, then transfer the cubes to an airtight container so you can take as many as you need at one time.

Per Serving (1 cup, made with coconut oil): Calories: 15; Total Fat: 2g; Cholesterol: 0mg; Sodium: 447mg; Carbs: 0g; Sugar: 0g; Fiber: 0g; Protein: 0g

Detoxifying Vegetable Soup

This soup is easy to digest and tastes wholesome and comforting. It can be eaten as part of a meal or for a delicious on-the-go snack.

Serves 8
PREP TIME: **10 minutes**
COOK TIME: **20 minutes**

2 cups chopped zucchini

½ pound green beans

½ cup chopped celery

2 tablespoons peeled and coarsely chopped fresh ginger

¼ cup fresh parsley leaves, plus ¼ cup chopped fresh parsley

2 quarts water

2 tablespoons coconut oil or organic grass-fed butter

1½ teaspoons sea salt

1. In a large soup pot over high heat, combine the zucchini, green beans, celery, ginger, parsley leaves, and water. Bring to a boil. Cover the pot and boil for about 15 minutes until the green beans are softened. Remove from the heat and add the coconut oil and salt.

2. Using an immersion blender, or working in batches in a standard blender, purée the soup until mostly smooth.

3. Stir in the chopped parsley and serve.

Make-ahead tip: Divide the soup among individual pint-size Mason jars for grab-and-go snacks or meals.

Per Serving (made with coconut oil): Calories: 47; Total Fat: 4g; Cholesterol: 0mg; Sodium: 452mg; Carbs: 3g; Sugar: 1g; Fiber: 1g; Protein: 1g

Pressure Cooker Bone Broth

Bone broth can be consumed year-round. In the summer, when it's hot, drinking warm beverages makes you sweat a little, in turn creating an evaporation process that cools you down. Bone broth is fairly easy to make once you get used to the process, but if just looking at this recipe is overwhelming, see the Resources section (page 206) for online sources to purchase a high-quality premade version.

Makes 6 cups

PREP TIME: **20 minutes**

COOK TIME: **2 hours**

2 pounds non-cartilaginous bones, such as marrow bones (no joint bones)

1 medium celery stalk, coarsely chopped

2 medium carrots, coarsely chopped

2 bay leaves

1 tablespoon peppercorns

3 fresh herb sprigs, such as parsley, rosemary, thyme, chives, or oregano, in any combination

2 tablespoons apple cider vinegar

1. Preheat the oven to 400°F.

2. Place the bones in a roasting pan and roast for 30 minutes.

3. Using oven-safe gloves or tongs, transfer the bones to a pressure cooker pot and add the celery, carrots, bay leaves, peppercorns, fresh herbs, and vinegar.

4. Fill the pot with water to 1 inch below the maximum fill line (about 6 cups). Lock the lid in place and close the pressure release valve. Select the Soup button and adjust the timer to 120 minutes.

5. Allow the pressure to release naturally after the cook time ends.

6. Remove the cooked vegetables and bones from the broth.

7. Strain the broth through a fine-mesh sieve to remove any smaller particles. Discard the solids. Transfer the broth to Mason jars and keep refrigerated for up to 4 days, or freeze.

SIBO tip: Using chicken bones or any joint or cartilaginous bones may produce a moderate- to high-FODMAP bone broth. However, some people don't react to a higher-FODMAP bone broth at all. If that's the case for you, feel free to make it with chicken bones or any joint bones.

Per Serving (1 cup): Calories: 90; Total Fat: 10g; Cholesterol: 45mg; Sodium: 120mg; Carbs: 2g; Sugar: 1g; Fiber: 1g; Protein: 15g

Puréed Zucchini Soup

For this zucchini soup, we peel the zucchini to make it easier to digest. If you're using larger zucchini with larger seeds, you can also remove the seeds as needed. For small to medium zucchini, you shouldn't need to remove them.

Serves 4

PREP TIME: **5 minutes**

COOK TIME: **20 minutes**

3 tablespoons organic grass-fed butter, ghee, or coconut oil

4 medium or 6 small zucchini, peeled, cut lengthwise, and sliced into half-moons

4 cups Low-FODMAP Vegetable Broth (page 90) or low-FODMAP chicken broth (see Resources, page 206)

Salt

Freshly ground black pepper

1. In a medium saucepan over medium-high heat, melt the butter.

2. Add the zucchini. Sauté for about 10 minutes, or until softened and beginning to brown.

3. Add the broth and bring to a boil. Reduce the heat to medium-low and simmer for 10 minutes. Using an immersion blender, or working in batches in a standard blender, carefully blend the soup until very smooth.

4. Season to taste with salt and pepper—the amount needed will depend on the amount of salt in the broth.

Preparation tip: If you prefer a vegan soup, use coconut oil and vegetable broth.

SIBO tip: Many people tolerate zucchini very well, so this is an easily digestible soup to nourish you if you're having increased symptoms.

Per Serving (made with butter and vegetable broth): Calories: 86; Total Fat: 7g; Cholesterol: 11mg; Sodium: 161mg; Carbs: 8g; Sugar: 4g; Fiber: 2g; Protein: 1g

Basic Carrot Soup

Carrots are an excellent source of vitamin A, biotin, and vitamins B_6, C, and K. This recipe is a great way to use extra carrots you don't want to throw out. Leave the scallion and celery out of the recipe if you're in the Calming Menu phase.

Serves 8

PREP TIME: **10 minutes**

COOK TIME: **40 minutes**

3 tablespoons organic grass-fed butter, ghee, or coconut oil

1 scallion, dark green parts only, chopped (optional)

1 celery stalk, chopped (optional)

5 cups chopped carrots or baby carrots

6 cups low-FODMAP chicken broth (see Resources, page 206) or Low-FODMAP Vegetable Broth (page 90)

Salt

1. In a heavy-bottomed saucepan over medium-high heat, melt the butter.

2. Add the scallion and celery (if using) and the carrots. Cook for 8 to 10 minutes, or until the vegetables are softened and beginning to brown.

3. Add the broth and bring to a low boil. Reduce the heat to medium-low and simmer for 20 to 25 minutes, or until the carrots are tender. Using an immersion blender, or working in batches in a standard blender, purée the soup until very smooth.

4. Season to taste with salt—the amount needed will depend on the amount of salt in the broth. Serve immediately or keep refrigerated.

Preparation tip: If you prefer a vegan soup, use coconut oil and vegetable broth.

Make-ahead tip: Double or triple this recipe and freeze for handy meals later.

Per Serving (made with vegetable broth and butter): Calories: 82; Total Fat: 7g; Cholesterol: 11mg; Sodium: 527mg; Carbs: 8g; Sugar: 4g; Fiber: 2g; Protein: 1g

Chicken and Rice Soup

This comforting soup is great during fall and winter and can be easily frozen and reheated.

Serves 4

PREP TIME: **10 minutes**

COOK TIME: **40 minutes**

2 tablespoons ghee, organic grass-fed butter, or coconut oil

¼ cup chopped scallion, dark green parts only

1 teaspoon dried Italian seasoning (without garlic)

⅓ cup chopped celery

1 cup chopped carrot

⅓ cup uncooked white rice

8 cups low-FODMAP chicken broth (see Resources, page 206)

2 cups cubed or shredded cooked organic chicken

1. In a large saucepan over medium-high heat, melt the ghee.

2. Add the scallion. Cook for about 3 minutes, or until softened.

3. Add the Italian seasoning, celery, and carrot. Cook for 4 minutes more, or until the vegetables begin to caramelize, stirring occasionally to avoid burning.

4. Add the rice and cook for 1 minute.

5. Stir in the chicken broth. Bring the soup to a boil. Cover the pot and reduce the heat to medium-low. Simmer for 20 minutes, or until the rice and vegetables are tender.

6. Add the chicken and simmer for 10 minutes more. Serve immediately or keep refrigerated.

Ingredient tip: There's truth to the myth . . . some scientists believe chicken soup may be more helpful than over-the-counter medications in dealing with a cold. When compared to warm water, eating chicken soup did a better job at moving nasal mucus.

Per Serving (made with ghee): Calories: 317; Total Fat: 9g; Cholesterol: 0mg; Sodium: 430mg; Carbs: 19g; Sugar: 2g; Fiber: 1g; Protein: 47g

Moroccan Carrot Soup

Moroccan spices give this simple carrot soup an interesting twist. Carrots are a good source of beta-carotene, vitamin K, potassium, and antioxidants.

Serves 4

PREP TIME: **10 minutes**

COOK TIME: **30 minutes**

½ cup 24-Hour Yogurt (page 84)

1 teaspoon ground cumin

2 tablespoons organic grass-fed butter or ghee

3 scallions, dark green parts only, sliced

1 pound carrots, diced, or 1 pound baby carrots

2½ cups low-FODMAP chicken broth (see Resources, page 206) or Low-FODMAP Vegetable Broth (page 90)

1 tablespoon pasteurized clover honey

1 teaspoon freshly squeezed lemon juice

⅛ teaspoon ground allspice

1. In a small bowl, stir together the yogurt and cumin. Set aside.

2. In a medium soup pot over medium-high heat, melt the butter.

3. Add the scallions. Sauté for 2 minutes.

4. Add the carrots. Sauté for 4 minutes.

5. Add the broth and bring the soup to a boil. Reduce the heat to medium-low and simmer for about 20 minutes, or until the carrots are tender. Remove the soup from the heat.

6. Using an immersion blender, or working in batches in a standard blender, purée the soup until smooth.

7. Whisk in the honey, lemon juice, and allspice.

8. Ladle the soup into four bowls and top each with a dollop of cumin yogurt.

Substitution tip: Use coconut cream instead of yogurt if you don't tolerate dairy.

Per Serving (made with butter and chicken broth): Calories: 175; Total Fat: 5g; Cholesterol: 20mg; Sodium: 255mg; Carbs: 19g; Sugar: 11g; Fiber: 3g; Protein: 10g

Sweet Potato Chili

Using bone broth gives this chili extra depth of flavor and makes it a nutrient-dense bowl of deliciousness.

Serves 6
PREP TIME: **10 minutes**
COOK TIME: **1 hour**

2 bay leaves

1 tablespoon ground cumin

1½ teaspoons sea salt

1 teaspoon chili powder

½ teaspoon dried oregano

½ teaspoon ground cinnamon

¼ teaspoon ground ginger

¼ teaspoon ground allspice

1 tablespoon ghee, organic grass-fed butter, or coconut oil

2 pounds grass-fed ground beef or turkey

2 cups crushed organic tomatoes or tomato sauce (without garlic)

2 cups Pressure Cooker Bone Broth (page 92)

3 cups cubed (bite-size) sweet potatoes

½ cup chopped celery

1 small avocado, pitted, peeled, and cut into eighths

3 tablespoons chopped fresh cilantro

1. In a small bowl, combine the bay leaves, cumin, salt, chili powder, oregano, cinnamon, ginger, and allspice. Set aside.

2. Heat the ghee in a large saucepan over medium heat.

3. Add the ground beef. Cook for about 10 minutes, or until browned and completely cooked through.

4. Pour in the tomatoes and bone broth and add the spice mixture. Stir, cover the pan, and simmer the chili for 5 minutes.

5. Add the sweet potatoes and celery. Re-cover the pan, reduce the heat to low, and simmer for 40 minutes. Serve in bowls, each topped with one-eighth of the avocado (you'll have two slices leftover) and a sprinkle of cilantro.

Substitution tip: Kabocha squash, also known as Japanese pumpkin, can be substituted for the sweet potatoes.

Per Serving (made with ghee and ground beef): Calories: 401; Total Fat: 20g; Cholesterol: 100mg; Sodium: 618mg; Carbs: 19g; Sugar: 5g; Fiber: 4g; Protein: 33g

Chilled Tomato Soup

This tomato soup makes a beautiful and delicious first course for a dinner party or can be part of an easy lunch at the office.

Serves 6

PREP TIME: **20 minutes, plus 1 hour to chill**

4 large organic tomatoes, diced

½ cucumber, peeled, seeded, and diced

½ organic red bell pepper, diced

2 tablespoons garlic oil

1 tablespoon apple cider vinegar

¾ teaspoon sea salt, plus more for seasoning if necessary

½ teaspoon ground cumin

⅛ teaspoon cayenne pepper (optional)

Freshly ground black pepper

1 medium avocado, pitted, peeled, and cut into six slices

2 tablespoons chopped fresh cilantro

½ cup 24-Hour Yogurt (page 84; optional)

1. In a blender, combine the tomatoes, cucumber, red bell pepper, garlic oil, vinegar, salt, cumin, and cayenne (if using). Blend until creamy. Season with more salt (if needed) and pepper to taste.

2. Refrigerate for at least 1 hour.

3. Ladle the soup into six bowls and top each with a slice of avocado, a sprinkle of cilantro, and a dollop of yogurt (if using).

Preparation tip: If you prefer a vegan soup, omit the yogurt.

Ingredient tip: As this recipe is relatively simple, the quality of the tomatoes shines through. When possible, buy fresh organic tomatoes from the farmers' market or grow your own at home!

Per Serving (made with cayenne pepper and yogurt): Calories: 120; Total Fat: 9g; Cholesterol: 1mg; Sodium: 231mg; Carbs: 9g; Sugar: 5g; Fiber: 4g; Protein: 2g

Orange and Olive Salad

This is a side salad for when you are able to digest some raw foods. Choose lettuces that are soft to the touch as they're easier to digest.

Serves 2

PREP TIME: **10 minutes**

2 cups soft organic lettuce, such as baby greens or butter lettuce

2 large oranges, peeled and segmented (see Tip below)

⅓ cup Kalamata or Picholine olives, pitted and halved

2 to 3 tablespoons Mustard Vinaigrette (page 196)

1 teaspoon chopped fresh parsley

1. Divide the lettuce between two small plates.

2. In a small bowl, combine the orange segments and olives.

3. Add the vinaigrette to the bowl and mix to coat the olives and oranges.

4. Top the lettuce with the orange and olive mixture. Sprinkle with the parsley and serve.

Technique tip: If you've never segmented an orange to remove the pith, it's not hard and there are numerous instructional videos on the Internet.

Per Serving: Calories: 465; Total Fat: 40g; Cholesterol: 0mg; Sodium: 120mg; Carbs: 27g; Sugar: 12g; Fiber: 5g; Protein: 3g

Cucumber, Tomato, and Yogurt Salad

This tangy salad includes healthy probiotics from the yogurt. It can be served immediately, or the yogurt sauce can be kept separately in the refrigerator until the salad is ready to be mixed and served.

Serves 4

PREP TIME: **15 minutes**

½ cup 24-Hour Yogurt (page 84)

2 tablespoons chopped fresh parsley

1 tablespoon chopped fresh cilantro

1 teaspoon ground cumin

1½ teaspoons freshly squeezed lemon juice

1 teaspoon lemon zest

Salt

Freshly ground black pepper

2 medium tomatoes, chopped and drained

2 medium cucumbers, peeled and seeded

1 cup shredded carrot

1. In a medium bowl, combine the yogurt, parsley, cilantro, cumin, lemon juice, and lemon zest. Whisk to combine. Season to taste with salt and pepper.

2. Add the tomatoes, cucumbers, and carrot. Gently stir to combine and serve immediately.

Substitution tip: If you don't tolerate yogurt, dress this salad with Mustard Vinaigrette (page 196) instead.

Per Serving: Calories: 46; Total Fat: 1g; Cholesterol: 3mg; Sodium: 41mg; Carbs: 7g; Sugar: 4g; Fiber: 2g; Protein: 2g

Fruit Salad with Mint-Lime Dressing

The bounty of summer is evident in this simple yet delicious fruit salad. Berries offer a host of nutrients and antioxidants, but any low-FODMAP fruit can be used. As fruit is the star of the show, buying organic instead of conventionally grown means reducing your pesticide exposure.

Serves 4

PREP TIME: **10 minutes**

¼ cup freshly squeezed lime juice

¼ cup pasteurized clover honey

¼ cup finely chopped
    fresh mint leaves

1 cup organic blueberries

1 cup organic strawberries

1 cup organic raspberries

1 cup halved organic grapes

1. In a medium bowl, whisk the lime juice and honey until incorporated.

2. Stir in the mint.

3. Add the fruit to the bowl and gently stir to combine. Serve immediately or keep refrigerated.

Substitution tip: If you don't like or tolerate mint, substitute fresh cilantro or basil.

Per Serving: Calories: 127; Total Fat: 0g; Cholesterol: 0mg; Sodium: 2mg; Carbs: 31g; Sugar: 25g; Fiber: 4g; Protein: 1g

Chicken Caesar Salad

If you tend to be very sensitive and are having many symptoms, it is best to buy a block of Parmesan cheese and grate it yourself as the pre-shredded and bagged cheeses tend to include anticaking agents that are not well tolerated by some people. Freshly grated tastes better, too.

Serves 1

PREP TIME: **10 minutes**

2 cups torn romaine lettuce leaves

2 tablespoons Caesar Salad Dressing (page 197)

1 cup shredded or cubed roast organic chicken

2 tablespoons finely grated Parmesan cheese

1 large hardboiled egg, sliced (optional)

1. Place the lettuce in a bowl or on a plate and add the dressing, making sure to coat all the leaves.

2. Scatter the chicken and sprinkle the Parmesan cheese over the lettuce.

3. If desired, top the salad with the hardboiled egg.

Make-ahead tip: This is a great salad to assemble the night before and take for lunch. Keep the dressing separate until ready to eat.

Per Serving: Calories: 425; Total Fat: 29g; Cholesterol: 342mg; Sodium: 491mg; Carbs: 1g; Sugar: 1g; Fiber: 1g; Protein: 36g

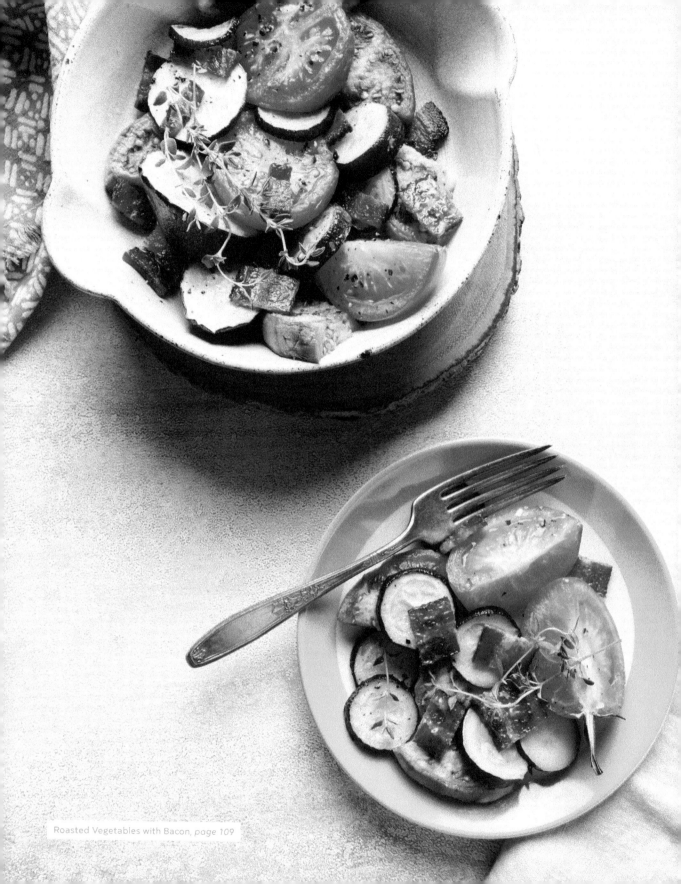

Roasted Vegetables with Bacon, *page 109*

Vegetables

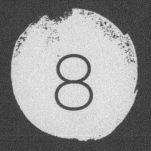

8

Carrot-Ginger Purée

This is a great basic recipe for those with leaky gut, as peeled and puréed veggies are easier to digest. If you don't care for ginger, try another savory spice like curry or cumin, or a sweet spice like cinnamon.

Serves 4

PREP TIME: **5 minutes**

COOK TIME: **20 minutes**

4 cups peeled and chopped carrots or baby carrots

3 tablespoons coconut oil, extra-virgin olive oil, organic grass-fed butter, or ghee

1 tablespoon peeled and chopped fresh ginger

Salt

Freshly ground black pepper

1. Steam the carrots for about 20 minutes until they are soft but not overly mushy. Transfer to a food processor.

2. Add the coconut oil and ginger. Blend until the carrots are puréed.

3. Season to taste with salt and pepper.

Variation tip: Blend this purée with Pressure Cooker Bone Broth (page 92) or Low-FODMAP Vegetable Broth (page 90) to make an easy, comforting soup.

Per Serving (made with coconut oil): Calories: 162; Total Fat: 11g; Cholesterol: 0mg; Sodium: 130mg; Carbs: 16g; Sugar: 10g; Fiber: 4g; Protein: 2g

Sautéed Spinach

Sautéed spinach is an incredibly easy side dish to make anytime. Spinach packs a nutritional punch as an excellent source of vitamins A, B2, B6, C, E, and K, manganese, folate, magnesium, iron, copper, calcium, and potassium!

Serves 1
PREP TIME: **5 minutes**
COOK TIME: **5 minutes**

1 tablespoon ghee, organic grass-fed butter, coconut oil, or bacon fat

1 to 2 cups fresh spinach

Salt

Freshly ground black pepper

1. In a medium or large skillet over high heat, melt the ghee.

2. When hot, add the spinach. Sauté, stirring, for about 2 minutes, or until wilted and soft.

3. Season to taste with salt and pepper. Serve immediately.

Preparation tip: If you prefer a vegan dish, use coconut oil.

Ingredient tip: In addition to using this vegetable as a side dish, throwing a handful of chopped raw spinach into scrambled eggs, soups, or stews increases the nutrient density of your meal.

Per Serving (made with ghee): Calories: 149; Total Fat: 15g; Cholesterol: 0mg; Sodium: 47mg; Carbs: 2g; Sugar: 0g; Fiber: 1g; Protein: 2g

Honey-Mustard Green Beans

Green beans contain a host of phytonutrients that act as anti-inflammatory agents.

Serves 6

PREP TIME: **5 minutes**

COOK TIME: **15 minutes**

3 tablespoons pasteurized clover honey

2 tablespoons Dijon or yellow mustard (without garlic)

¼ teaspoon sea salt, plus more for seasoning

1 pound fresh green beans

6 bacon slices, chopped

Freshly ground black pepper

1. In a small bowl, stir together the honey, mustard, and salt. Set aside.

2. Add the green beans to a medium saucepan filled with water and bring to a boil over high heat. Cook for about 10 minutes, or until very tender.

3. While the green beans boil, in a large skillet over medium heat, cook the bacon until slightly crispy. Set the skillet aside until the green beans are done. Drain the green beans in a colander.

4. Return the skillet with the bacon to medium-high heat. Add the cooked green beans and honey-mustard sauce. Sauté the green beans with the bacon and sauce for 5 minutes.

5. Season to taste with salt and pepper. Serve immediately.

Preparation tip: To make this dish vegetarian, omit the bacon and add 1 teaspoon coconut oil to the skillet when sautéing the green beans with the sauce.

Per Serving: Calories: 99; Total Fat: 4g; Cholesterol: 8mg; Sodium: 199mg; Carbs: 13g; Sugar: 9g; Fiber: 1g; Protein: 4g

Roasted Vegetables with Bacon

Not only do these vegetables make a great side dish, but they can also be topped with a fried egg or leftover chicken for a delicious breakfast or lunch the next day.

Serves 4
PREP TIME: **15 minutes**
COOK TIME: **40 minutes**

4 large organic plum tomatoes, coarsely chopped or cut into wedges

2 large zucchini, sliced

1 medium eggplant, peeled and sliced

1 tablespoon coconut oil, melted

8 bacon slices

1 tablespoon garlic oil

Salt

Freshly ground black pepper

1. Preheat the oven to 375°F. Line a rimmed baking sheet with parchment paper.

2. Place the tomatoes, zucchini, and eggplant on the prepared sheet. Add the coconut oil and toss to coat. Bake for about 40 minutes, or until all the vegetables are softened.

3. Meanwhile, in a large skillet over medium heat, cook the bacon. Transfer to paper towels to drain. When the bacon is cool enough to handle, chop it into bite-size pieces.

4. Remove the vegetables from the oven and mix in the bacon and garlic oil.

5. Season to taste with salt and pepper. Serve warm or at room temperature.

Ingredient tip: Tomatoes are in the nightshade family and may cause inflammation in some people. Interestingly, though, several research studies have actually linked tomatoes to decreased inflammation and oxidative stress. So make your own judgment about tomatoes and how they affect you.

Per Serving: Calories: 200; Total Fat: 14g; Cholesterol: 20mg; Sodium: 365mg; Carbs: 12g; Sugar: 9g; Fiber: 6g; Protein: 10g

Baked Eggplant

The garlic oil in this baked eggplant combined with parsley will give you the aromas and taste you've been missing.

Serves 2

PREP TIME: **10 minutes**

COOK TIME: **30 minutes**

2 small eggplants, halved
   lengthwise

3 tablespoons finely
   chopped fresh parsley

3 tablespoons garlic oil

Salt

Freshly ground black pepper

1. Preheat the oven to 350°F. Line a rimmed baking sheet with parchment paper.

2. Using a sharp knife, make horizontal and vertical cuts about two-thirds deep into each eggplant half, forming a checkerboard.

3. Insert the chopped parsley inside the cuts in the eggplant. Put the eggplant halves on the prepared sheet.

4. Drizzle the garlic oil over the eggplant and sprinkle generously with salt and pepper.

5. Bake for about 30 minutes, or until the eggplant is softened.

SIBO tip: Eggplant is a very good source of fiber, but if you don't digest higher-fiber foods well, avoid eating the skin.

Per Serving: Calories: 297; Total Fat: 22g; Cholesterol: 0mg; Sodium: 12mg; Carbs: 27g; Sugar: 16g; Fiber: 14g; Protein: 5g

Balsamic Green Beans

The cooking method for these green beans makes them tender and easily digestible. Larger servings (more than 17 whole beans) contain moderate amounts of the FODMAP sorbitol, so limit your consumption as needed.

Serves 4
PREP TIME: **10 minutes**
COOK TIME: **40 minutes**

1 pound green beans, trimmed

2 tablespoons avocado oil

2 scallions, dark green parts only, chopped

1 bay leaf

4 cups low-FODMAP chicken broth (see Resources, page 206) or Low-FODMAP Vegetable Broth (page 90)

2 tablespoons aged balsamic vinegar

2 tablespoons extra-virgin olive oil

Salt

Freshly ground black pepper

1. Bring a large pot of water to a boil over high heat. Add the green beans and cook for about 5 minutes, or until crisp-tender. Drain and set aside.

2. Heat the avocado oil in a large saucepan over medium-high heat until hot but not smoking.

3. Add the scallions and bay leaf. Sauté for about 3 minutes, stirring occasionally until soft.

4. Add the green beans, chicken broth, vinegar, and olive oil. Bring the mixture to a simmer. Reduce the heat to low, cover the pan, and simmer for 25 minutes.

5. Remove the lid and simmer for about 5 minutes more, or until the remaining liquid is reduced.

6. Remove and discard the bay leaf. Season the green beans to taste with salt and pepper. Serve immediately.

Preparation tip: If you prefer a vegan dish, use vegetable broth.

SIBO tip: Lower-quality balsamic vinegars can sometimes have added sugar that some people may not tolerate. Look for aged balsamic vinegar and double-check the ingredients label.

Per Serving: Calories: 187; Total Fat: 14g; Cholesterol: 0mg; Sodium: 114mg; Carbs: 10g; Sugar: 5g; Fiber: 3g; Protein: 4g

Curried Bok Choy

Adding a little curry powder to this bok choy makes it interesting without being overly spicy. Curry powder contains turmeric, which has anti-inflammatory properties.

Serves 4

PREP TIME: **10 minutes**

COOK TIME: **20 minutes**

1 tablespoon coconut oil

2 tablespoons yellow curry powder

¼ teaspoon sea salt

½ teaspoon red pepper flakes (optional)

1 large bok choy, or 3 or 4 baby bok choy, cut into bite-size pieces, stems and leaves separated

1 (13.5-ounce) can coconut milk (BPA- and gum-free, if possible)

2 teaspoons freshly squeezed lime juice

½ cup chopped fresh cilantro

1. In a medium skillet or sauté pan over medium heat, melt the coconut oil.

2. Stir in the curry powder, salt, and red pepper flakes (if using). Cook for about 1 minute.

3. Place the bok choy stems evenly over the bottom of the pan and layer the leaves on top. Pour the coconut milk over the bok choy. Cover the skillet and reduce the heat to medium-low. Simmer for 10 to 15 minutes, or until the stems are tender and the leaves are wilted.

4. Remove the skillet from the heat and stir in the lime juice and cilantro. Serve warm.

Preparation tip: Serve this curried bok choy over white rice or with an added protein, such as chicken, to make a meal.

Per Serving: Calories: 214; Total Fat: 22g; Cholesterol: 0mg; Sodium: 204mg; Carbs: 6g; Sugar: 2g; Fiber: 0g; Protein: 2g

Tender Swiss Chard

If you are having multiple symptoms and digestion issues, it's best to remove the ribs of the chard because they are rough and can be hard to digest.

Serves 2 to 4
PREP TIME: **10 minutes**
COOK TIME: **35 minutes**

2 tablespoons coconut oil

2 bunches Swiss chard, ribs and leaves separated and coarsely chopped

1½ teaspoons garlic oil

Salt

Freshly ground black pepper

1. In a large skillet over medium-high heat, melt the coconut oil.

2. Add the chard ribs to the skillet. Sauté for about 5 minutes, or until softened.

3. Add the chard leaves and cover the skillet. Reduce the heat to medium and cook for 10 to 15 minutes, or until the greens are tender and wilted.

4. Add the garlic oil and season to taste with salt and pepper. Stir to combine.

5. Reduce the heat to low and cook for 10 minutes more. Serve hot.

Ingredient tip: Swiss chard hasn't gotten as much positive press as kale, but it is a nutrient powerhouse with excellent levels of vitamins A, C, E, and K, as well as magnesium, copper, and iron.

Per Serving (1 cup): Calories: 195; Total Fat: 18g; Cholesterol: 0mg; Sodium: 510mg; Carbs: 10g; Sugar: 5g; Fiber: 5g; Protein: 5g

Zucchini Chips

Zucchini chips are a great option when you want a crispy, salty treat. Just one zucchini has 50 percent of the daily recommended intake of vitamin C! Snack on.

Serves 4

PREP TIME: **10 minutes**

COOK TIME: **2 to 3 hours**

4 cups very thinly sliced zucchini (from 2 or 3 medium zucchini; use a mandoline or very sharp knife)

2 tablespoons coconut oil or ghee, melted

2 teaspoons coarse sea salt

1. Preheat the oven to 200°F (see Tip below). Line a baking sheet with parchment paper.

2. In a large bowl, combine the zucchini and coconut oil. Toss to coat. Place the zucchini evenly on the prepared sheet and sprinkle with the salt. Bake for 2 to 3 hours, or until the chips are crispy, rotating the pan halfway through cooking.

3. Let the chips cool and store in an airtight glass container.

Preparation tip: You can increase the oven temperature to reduce cooking time, but check the oven frequently to avoid burning the zucchini.

Per Serving: Calories: 85; Total Fat: 7g; Cholesterol: 0mg; Sodium: 1,172mg; Carbs: 5g; Sugar: 4g; Fiber: 2g; Protein: 2g

Kale Chips

If you don't know already, you'll be surprised by how delicious and addictive kale chips are! After you separate the kale leaves from the ribs, the ribs can be frozen for use in Low-FODMAP Vegetable Broth (page 90).

Serves 2

PREP TIME: **10 minutes**

COOK TIME: **15 minutes**

2 bunches kale, washed and thoroughly dried

2 tablespoons coconut aminos

2 tablespoons extra-virgin olive or avocado oil

1. Preheat the oven to 350°F. Line a baking sheet with parchment paper.

2. Using kitchen shears or tearing by hand, remove the kale leaves from the ribs and tear into bite-size pieces. Place the kale on the prepared sheet.

3. Pour the coconut aminos and olive oil over the kale and, using clean hands, massage into the kale. Bake the chips for 12 to 15 minutes. They should be crispy, not chewy, so some leaves may need to stay in the oven longer than others.

4. Serve the kale chips immediately, or let cool and store in an airtight glass container. If they get soft, they can be crisped up in a 350°F oven for a couple of minutes.

Ingredient tip: If you don't like or can't tolerate coconut aminos, omit this ingredient and lightly salt the kale chips before baking instead. Limit the amount of salt you use, because the leaves will shrink as they cook, and you'll end up with a fair amount of salt on a small piece of kale.

Per Serving (made with extra-virgin olive oil): Calories: 270; Total Fat: 15g; Cholesterol: 0mg; Sodium: 270mg; Carbs: 23g; Sugar: 3g; Fiber: 0g; Protein: 9g

Broccoli with Lemon-Mustard Butter

Broccoli has antioxidant, anti-inflammatory, and detoxification components that make it a great choice for your weekly menu.

Serves 2 or 3, depending on the size of the broccoli

PREP TIME: **5 minutes**

COOK TIME: **30 minutes**

1 tablespoon ghee or coconut oil

1 large head broccoli (florets only), cut into bite-size pieces

Salt

6 tablespoons organic grass-fed butter

2 tablespoons freshly squeezed lemon juice

2 tablespoons Dijon or regular mustard (without garlic)

1 teaspoon lemon zest

1. Preheat the oven to 400°F. Grease a baking sheet with the ghee.

2. Arrange the broccoli in a single layer on the prepared sheet. Sprinkle lightly with salt. Roast the broccoli for about 15 minutes, or until it begins to soften.

3. Meanwhile, in a small saucepan over medium heat, melt the butter.

4. Whisk in the lemon juice, mustard, and lemon zest.

5. Remove the broccoli from the oven and spoon the lemon-mustard butter over it, stirring to coat. Return the broccoli to the oven and cook for 10 to 15 minutes more, or until softened. Serve immediately.

SIBO tip: For those who do well with cruciferous vegetables, this recipe can be introduced in Week 1. If you don't know whether you tolerate broccoli, wait until Week 4 and start with a smaller portion. Broccoli stalks contain higher concentrations of FODMAPs, which is why this recipe uses florets only.

Per Serving: Calories: 278; Total Fat: 28g; Cholesterol: 61mg; Sodium: 420mg; Carbs: 4g; Sugar: 1g; Fiber: 1g; Protein: 2g

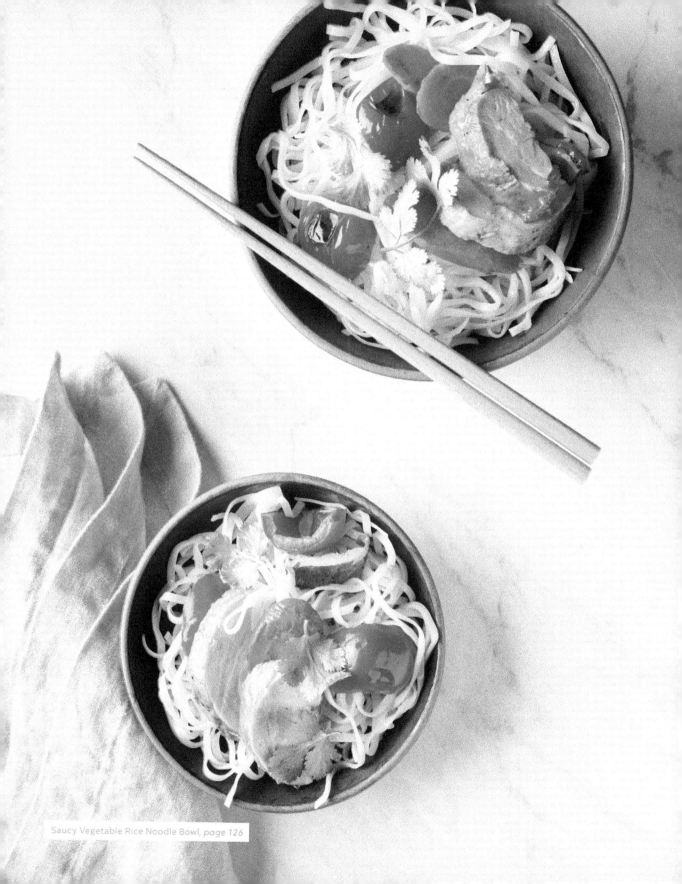

Saucy Vegetable Rice Noodle Bowl, *page 126*

Potatoes and Grains

Basic White Rice

White rice is included early on in the meal plan, as it tends to be very easy to digest. If you haven't been incorporating rice or other grains into your diet, start with a small serving of ¼ cup and increase to ½ cup to 1 cup as tolerated.

Serves 4

PREP TIME: **5 minutes**

COOK TIME: **20 minutes**

2 cups water or Pressure Cooker Bone Broth (page 92)

2 tablespoons ghee, organic grass-fed butter, or coconut oil

1 teaspoon sea salt

1 cup white rice

1. In a medium saucepan with a lid over high heat, bring the water and salt to a boil.

2. Add the rice and stir. Cover the pan and reduce the heat to medium-low. Cook for 20 minutes without uncovering.

3. Remove from the heat, uncover, and fluff the rice with the fork. If any water remains or if the rice isn't fully cooked, return the pan to the still-warm burner until the water evaporates and the rice is cooked.

4. Stir in the ghee, butter, or coconut oil and serve.

Preparation tip: If you prefer a vegan rice, use water and coconut oil.

Ingredient tip: Replace the water or broth with coconut milk to make a delicious coconut rice.

Per Serving: Calories: 225; Total Fat: 7g; Cholesterol: 16mg; Sodium: 442mg; Carbs: 37g; Sugar: 0g; Fiber: 1g; Protein: 3g

Herbed Rice

White rice is included in the diet early on because it is low-FODMAP and low-fiber, making it easily digestible. However, it may cause symptoms in people who can't tolerate starch. If that happens, remove it from your diet and try it again in a smaller portion in a couple of weeks. If you prefer a paleo diet, substitute bone broth or a second vegetable for the rice in a meal.

Serves 4
PREP TIME: **5 minutes**
COOK TIME: **25 minutes**

3 tablespoons unsalted organic grass-fed butter, ghee, or coconut oil

1 cup white rice

1 small bunch fresh chives, chopped

1 tablespoon fresh thyme leaves

2 cups low-FODMAP chicken broth (see Resources, page 206), Low-FODMAP Vegetable Broth (page 90), or Pressure Cooker Bone Broth (page 92)

2 tablespoons fresh parsley leaves

Salt

Freshly ground black pepper

1. In a medium saucepan over medium heat, melt the butter.

2. Add the rice, chives, and thyme. Sauté for about 4 minutes, or until the herbs are softened.

3. Pour the broth over the rice, stir, and cover the pan. Reduce the heat to medium-low and cook for about 15 minutes, or until the rice is tender.

4. Stir in the parsley. Season to taste with salt and pepper. Let it sit for 5 minutes and serve.

SIBO tip: Chives or scallions (dark green parts only) often substitute for onions on a SIBO diet. Chives provide a more delicate flavor than scallions.

Per Serving (made with butter): Calories: 173; Total Fat: 10g; Cholesterol: 23mg; Sodium: 127mg; Carbs: 15g; Sugar: 0g; Fiber: 1g; Protein: 61g

Buttery Rice Noodles

This simple rice dish is great when you need some added carbohydrates but are reacting to many vegetables. You can also add any vegetables you can tolerate.

Serves 4

PREP TIME: **10 minutes**

COOK TIME: **10 minutes**

1 (8-ounce) package white rice noodles (see Tip below)

⅓ cup organic grass-fed butter or ghee

Salt

Freshly ground black pepper

2 tablespoons fresh parsley leaves (optional)

1. Cook the rice noodles according to package instructions. Drain in a colander and transfer to a medium bowl.

2. Stir the butter into the hot noodles, allowing it to melt and coat the noodles.

3. Season to taste with salt and pepper. Sprinkle with parsley (if using) and serve.

Ingredient tip: Rice noodles can be found in most supermarkets and in Asian food markets. Make sure the only ingredients are either white rice or white rice flour and water.

Per Serving (made with butter): Calories: 340; Total Fat: 15g; Cholesterol: 40mg; Sodium: 225mg; Carbs: 47g; Sugar: 0g; Fiber: 0g; Protein: 2g

Dilly Potato Salad

Many people with SIBO tolerate peeled white potatoes as a starch in their diet. Because it's high-glycemic, it absorbs quickly and typically doesn't cause symptoms, but it's always good to pair it with a fat so it doesn't cause a blood sugar spike. Here we pair it with a healthy olive oil as part of this delicious salad.

Serves 6

PREP TIME: **10 minutes**

COOK TIME: **20 minutes**

2 pounds red potatoes, peeled and halved

½ cup extra-virgin olive oil

⅓ cup apple cider vinegar

1 tablespoon mustard (without garlic)

2 scallions, dark green parts only, sliced

2 tablespoons chopped fresh dill

Salt

Freshly ground black pepper

1. Put the potatoes in a large saucepan and fully cover them with salted cold water. Place the pan over high heat and bring to a boil. Cook for 10 to 15 minutes, or until tender. Remove from the heat, drain, and transfer to a large bowl.

2. In a small bowl, whisk the olive oil, vinegar, and mustard. Add the dressing to the potatoes along with the scallions and dill. Mix everything together and season to taste with salt and pepper. Serve warm or cold.

Preparation tip: Add chopped cooked bacon if you're a bacon lover.

Substitution tip: If you don't like dill, substitute tarragon or another fresh herb instead.

Per Serving: Calories: 269; Total Fat: 18g; Cholesterol: 0mg; Sodium: 147mg; Carbs: 21g; Sugar: 2g; Fiber: 3g; Protein: 3g

Creamy Mashed Potatoes

Mashed potatoes are not only comfort food but also often work well for people with SIBO because they're low in fiber.

Serves 4

PREP TIME: **10 minutes**

COOK TIME: **20 minutes**

2 pounds organic white
russet potatoes, peeled

8 tablespoons ghee or
organic grass-fed butter
(1 stick), softened

⅔ cup lactose-free milk or other
milk of choice, warmed

1 teaspoon sea salt

2 tablespoons chopped
fresh chives

1. Put the potatoes in a large pot and fully cover them with cold water. Place the pot over high heat and bring to a boil. Reduce the heat to medium-high and cook for 20 minutes, or until the potatoes are soft and easily pierced with a fork. Drain, transfer to a large bowl, and add the ghee.

2. Using a handheld electric mixer with the whisk attachment, start to break up the potatoes while adding the warm milk.

3. Add the salt and mix until smooth. Serve topped with the chives.

Preparation tip: For a dairy-free version, use coconut oil and nut or coconut milk.

Per Serving (made with ghee): Calories: 585; Total Fat: 31g; Cholesterol: 3mg; Sodium: 462mg; Carbs: 71g; Sugar: 6g; Fiber: 5g; Protein: 9g

Sweet Potato Wedges

Try different spices in this recipe to find your favorite. Use Chinese five-spice powder for a sweeter flavor, or paprika or chili powder for a spicy kick. These wedges are a delicious accompaniment for any meal of the day.

Serves 4

PREP TIME: **10 minutes**

COOK TIME: **30 minutes**

2 medium sweet potatoes, peeled, halved lengthwise, and cut into small wedges

1 tablespoon garlic oil, melted coconut oil, organic grass-fed butter, or ghee

1 teaspoon ground cumin

1 teaspoon sea salt

¼ teaspoon freshly ground black pepper

Low-FODMAP ketchup or low-FODMAP Ranch Dressing (page 198), for dipping

1. Preheat the oven to 425°F.

2. On a rimmed baking sheet, toss the sweet potato wedges with the garlic oil, cumin, salt, and pepper. Arrange in a single layer.

3. Roast for about 30 minutes, or until the wedges are tender and browned. Serve immediately with ketchup or ranch dressing for dipping.

SIBO tip: Peeling the sweet potatoes makes them easier to digest. If you do well with fiber, leave the skin on.

Per Serving (without dipping sauce): Calories: 88; Total Fat: 4g; Cholesterol: 0mg; Sodium: 477mg; Carbs: 13g; Sugar: 4g; Fiber: 2g; Protein: 1g

Saucy Vegetable Rice Noodle Bowl

This rice noodle dish is an easy weeknight dinner, plus it's a great option to make ahead and take for lunch during the week.

Serves 2

PREP TIME: **15 minutes**

COOK TIME: **10 minutes**

1 tablespoon coconut oil

2 cups shredded or sliced carrots

1 organic red bell pepper, chopped or sliced

3 tablespoons rice wine vinegar

2 tablespoons extra-virgin olive oil

1 tablespoon garlic oil

2½ tablespoons almond or peanut butter

1½ tablespoons coconut aminos

1 tablespoon peeled and minced fresh ginger

3 ounces (1½ cups) white rice noodles

1½ cups shredded or cubed cooked organic chicken (optional)

¼ cup chopped fresh cilantro

1. In a large skillet over medium-high heat, melt the coconut oil.

2. When the oil is hot, add the carrots and red bell pepper. Cook, stirring occasionally, for about 10 minutes, or until the vegetables are softened.

3. In a small bowl, whisk the vinegar, olive oil, garlic oil, nut butter, coconut aminos, and ginger. Set aside.

4. Cook the rice noodles according to package instructions until softened. Drain and divide between two bowls. Top the noodles with the nut butter sauce, vegetables, and chicken (if using). Sprinkle with the cilantro and serve immediately.

Preparation tip: If you prefer a vegan or vegetarian meal, omit the chicken.

Ingredient tip: A study on organic bell peppers found them to have higher nutritional content than conventionally grown ones. Additionally, bell peppers are No. 6 on the Dirty Dozen list (see page 204), so buy them organic whenever possible.

Per Serving (made with almond butter): Calories: 717; Total Fat: 44g; Cholesterol: 0mg; Sodium: 408mg; Carbs: 59g; Sugar: 12g; Fiber: 6g; Protein: 31g

Vegetable-Herb Quinoa Salad

Feel free to add a protein like cooked chicken to this cold salad to make it a meal. This is a great dish to make at the beginning of the week and take for lunch.

Serves 4

PREP TIME: **30 minutes**

COOK TIME: **10 minutes**

2 cups quinoa, cooked according to package instructions

2 cups steamed broccoli crowns

2 cups organic cherry tomatoes, halved

1 cup shredded carrots, steamed or raw

¼ cup fresh basil leaves, chopped

2 tablespoons chopped fresh parsley leaves

2 tablespoons chopped fresh chives

⅔ cup extra-virgin olive oil

¼ cup white wine vinegar

1 heaping tablespoon regular or Dijon mustard (without garlic)

¼ cup microgreens

1. In a medium bowl, combine the cooked quinoa, steamed broccoli, tomatoes, carrots, basil, parsley, and chives.

2. In a blender, combine the olive oil, vinegar, and mustard. Blend until mixed well. Pour the dressing over the salad and stir to combine.

3. Top the salad with the microgreens. Serve immediately or keep refrigerated.

Ingredient tip: Microgreens might sound trendy, but a 2012 study showed that some microgreens have up to 40 percent more nutrients than their mature vegetable counterparts.

Per Serving (made with regular mustard): Calories: 529; Total Fat: 40g; Cholesterol: 0mg; Sodium: 263mg; Carbs: 37g; Sugar: 8g; Fiber: 11g; Protein: 12g

Curry Quinoa Stir-Fry

Use the vegetables noted in this recipe, or make your own combinations using whatever you have in your refrigerator. Just remember to start with vegetables that need to be cooked longer and then add the vegetables that require a shorter cooking time. You can also add more coconut milk for a saucier version, or more curry for a spicier version.

Serves 4

PREP TIME: **5 minutes**

COOK TIME: **20 minutes**

2 tablespoons coconut oil

1 cup shredded carrots

1 cup chopped fresh spinach

2 cups quinoa, cooked according to package instructions

2 cups chopped cooked organic chicken

2 teaspoons yellow curry powder

½ cup coconut milk

Salt

1. In a large saucepan over medium-high heat, melt the coconut oil.

2. Add the carrots. Sauté for 10 minutes, or until tender.

3. Add the spinach. Cook for 1 minute more.

4. Stir in the cooked quinoa and chicken, the curry powder, and coconut milk. Cook for 5 minutes, or until hot. Season to taste with salt and serve immediately.

Ingredient tip: Curry powder contains turmeric, which has been shown to have strong anti-inflammatory properties.

Per Serving: Calories: 308; Total Fat: 15g; Cholesterol: 0mg; Sodium: 42mg; Carbs: 24g; Sugar: 3g; Fiber: 4g; Protein: 24g

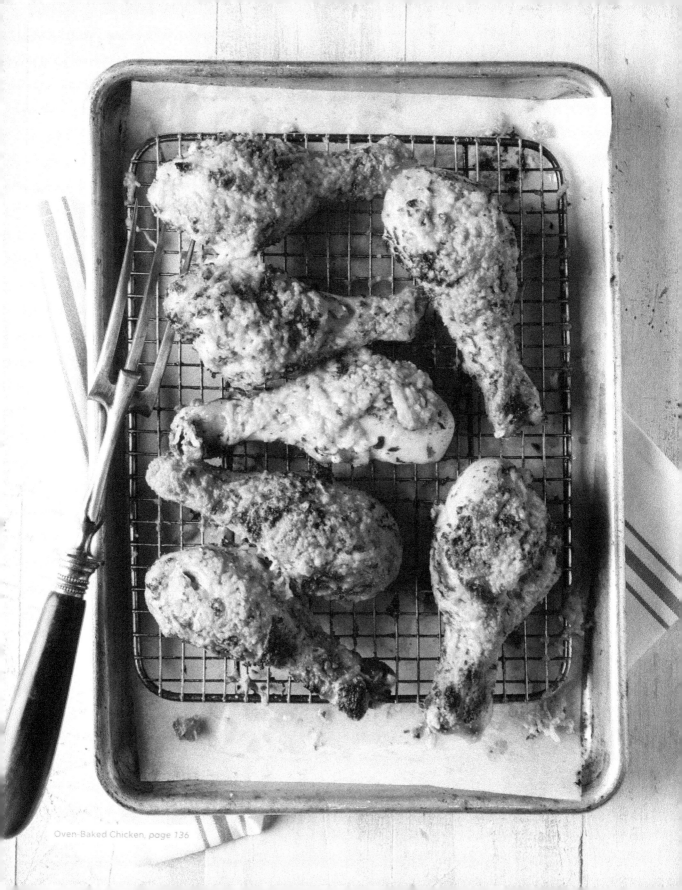

Oven-Baked Chicken, page 136

Poultry

Simple Roast Chicken

Luckily, roast chicken seasoned with only salt and pepper is available at many grocery stores. However, if you can take the time to make your own, you'll be rewarded with the taste (and smell) of freshly cooked chicken with crispy skin, hot from the oven.

Serves 4 to 6
PREP TIME: **10 minutes**
COOK TIME: **1 hour 10 minutes**

1 (2- to 3-pound) organic chicken

3 or 4 fresh or dried herb sprigs, including thyme, sage, or rosemary, for stuffing, plus 1 teaspoon fresh or dried herbs, including thyme, rosemary, or dried Italian seasoning (without garlic), for seasoning (all optional)

1 lemon, quartered (optional)

1 tablespoon coconut oil, unsalted organic grass-fed butter, or ghee, melted for brushing

Kosher salt or sea salt (such as Real Salt brand)

Freshly ground black pepper

1. Preheat the oven to 450°F.

2. Remove the chicken from its wrapping and pat dry with paper towels. Place in a roasting pan or on a rimmed baking sheet.

3. Stuff the chicken cavity with the herb sprigs and the lemon (if using), and truss the chicken, if desired (see Tip below).

4. Using your hands or a pastry brush, slather the chicken all over with the coconut oil.

5. Generously season the chicken on all sides with salt and pepper. Sprinkle the remaining 1 teaspoon of herbs (if using) over the chicken. Bake for 1 hour, or until fully cooked and the juices run clear.

6. Remove the chicken from the oven and let sit for 10 minutes before serving.

Technique tip: Trussing a chicken helps it cook more evenly. If you haven't trussed a chicken before, it's relatively easy—pictorial or video instructions can be found online.

Per Serving (made with a 2-pound chicken): Calories: 391; Total Fat: 24g; Cholesterol: 127.5mg; Sodium: 120mg; Carbs: 0g; Sugar: 0g; Fiber: 31.5g; Protein: 44g

Poached Chicken Breast

Poached chicken can be eaten alone, with a sauce like Romesco Sauce (page 199) or Chimichurri Sauce (page 195), on top of a salad, or as part of a bowl with grains and vegetables.

Serves 3

PREP TIME: **5 minutes**

COOK TIME: **35 minutes**

1 pound boneless, skinless organic chicken breasts

2 cups cold water

2 teaspoons Italian seasoning (without garlic) or herbes de Provence

2 bay leaves

1 organic lemon, sliced

1. Place the chicken breasts in a heavy-bottomed medium saucepan. Cover with the water and add the Italian seasoning, bay leaves, and lemon slices. Bring the mixture to a boil over high heat. Reduce the heat to low and partially cover the pan. Simmer for about 10 minutes.

2. Turn off the heat and leave the chicken breasts in the hot poaching liquid for 20 minutes.

3. Remove the chicken from the poaching liquid and let cool before slicing or shredding.

Technique tip: Chicken breasts are relatively low in fat, so poaching tends to leave them moister than other cooking methods.

Per Serving: Calories: 179; Total Fat: 4g; Cholesterol: 93mg; Sodium: 176mg; Carbs: 0g; Sugar: 0g; Fiber: 0g; Protein: 32g

Deli Meat Roll-Ups

It may seem strange at first to be eating these ingredients without bread, but deli meat roll-ups are extremely quick to put together and make a filling snack or meal.

Serves 1

PREP TIME: **5 minutes**

6 slices deli meat, such as organic turkey or roast beef

1½ teaspoons mustard (without garlic), for spreading

1½ teaspoons mayonnaise, for spreading

3 tablespoons organic microgreens

1 small tomato, chopped

3 bacon slices, cooked

3 small pieces avocado (one-eighth of an avocado)

1. On a work surface, overlap 2 slices of deli meat. Spread some of the mustard and mayonnaise on each piece.

2. Place 1 tablespoon of microgreens, one-third of the tomato, 1 bacon slice, and 1 piece of avocado in the center of the meat. Fold the meat in half, then fold it over again to create a roll. Repeat Steps 1 and 2 to make a total of three roll-ups.

3. Pack in a glass container for a meal on the go.

SIBO tip: Choose deli meat, mustard, and mayonnaise made without added garlic or onion. Microgreens are very tender and make a nutrient-dense addition to this quick meal.

Per Serving (made with turkey): Calories: 470; Total Fat: 26g; Cholesterol: 142mg; Sodium: 2,592mg; Carbs: 9g; Sugar: 7g; Fiber: 2g; Protein: 46g

Sautéed Chicken Livers

Chicken livers are loaded with vitamin B$_{12}$ and iron, both of which are often low in people with SIBO.

Serves 4

PREP TIME: **10 minutes**

COOK TIME: **10 minutes**

⅓ pound bacon

1 pound organic chicken
    livers, trimmed

¼ cup dry white wine

1 tablespoon aged
    balsamic vinegar

1 tablespoon drained capers

2 tablespoons chopped
    fresh flat-leaf parsley

1 tablespoon chopped chives

Salt

Freshly ground black pepper

1. In a large skillet over medium heat, cook the bacon until crisp. With a slotted spoon, transfer to a paper towel–lined plate to drain, leaving the bacon fat in the skillet. When the bacon is cool enough to handle, coarsely chop it.

2. Increase the heat to medium-high and, working in 2 batches, add the chicken livers to the skillet. Cook for 1½ to 2 minutes per side, or until browned. Transfer the livers to a plate.

3. Return the skillet to the heat and stir in the wine, vinegar, and capers, scraping up any browned bits from the bottom of the pan. Bring to a boil and cook for 1 minute until thickened slightly.

4. Stir in the parsley and chives.

5. Stir in the livers and bacon. Season to taste with salt and pepper.

Technique tip: Adding liquid to a pan, in this case white wine and balsamic vinegar, after browning meat or vegetables is called deglazing. The addition of the browned bits to the liquids, capers, parsley, and chives makes a delicious sauce.

Per Serving: Calories: 400; Total Fat: 20g; Cholesterol: 42mg; Sodium: 5,790mg; Carbs: 19g; Sugar: 3g; Fiber: 9g; Protein: 40g

Oven-Baked Chicken

This baked chicken has a delicious crispy crust while also being gluten-free.

Serves 6
PREP TIME: **10 minutes**
COOK TIME: **50 minutes**

3 pounds skin-on organic chicken, thighs, legs, or breasts

Salt

Freshly ground black pepper

1 cup white rice flour

½ teaspoon paprika (optional)

½ teaspoon Italian seasoning (without garlic)

1 tablespoon organic grass-fed butter, ghee, or coconut oil, melted

1 tablespoon garlic oil

1. Preheat the oven to 400°F. Line a baking sheet with parchment paper.

2. Pat the chicken dry with paper towels and generously season with salt and pepper.

3. In a gallon-size resealable plastic bag, combine the white rice flour, paprika (if using), and Italian seasoning. Seal the bag and shake to mix the flour and spices.

4. Add half of the chicken to the bag. Seal and shake to coat. Transfer the chicken to the prepared sheet. Repeat with the remaining chicken.

5. In a small bowl, stir together the butter and garlic oil. Drizzle the mixture over the chicken.

6. Bake for 50 minutes, or until done and the juices run clear.

SIBO tip: Gluten-free all-purpose flour can be substituted for the white rice flour in this recipe, but it often contains multiple ingredients, including gums, whereas white rice flour typically only includes rice, so you are more likely to tolerate it if you tolerate white rice.

Per Serving (made with chicken thighs and butter): Calories: 444; Total Fat: 27g; Cholesterol: 136mg; Sodium: 138mg; Carbs: 21g; Sugar: 0g Fiber: 1g; Protein: 29g

Garlic-Parmesan Chicken Legs

Feel free to substitute chicken thighs or wings for the chicken legs in this recipe. If you use chicken wings, this recipe makes an excellent appetizer.

Serves 4
PREP TIME: **5 minutes**
COOK TIME: **40 minutes**

1 tablespoon Italian seasoning (without garlic)

1 teaspoon ground cumin

½ teaspoon sea salt

2 pounds organic chicken legs

⅓ cup grated Parmesan cheese

2 tablespoons garlic oil

1. Preheat the oven to 425°F.

2. In a large bowl, mix together the Italian seasoning, cumin, and salt.

3. Pat the chicken legs dry with paper towels and toss them with the spice mixture, making sure they are evenly coated. Place the legs on a baking sheet. Cook for 35 minutes, or until cooked through and the juices run clear.

4. Turn the oven to broil, and broil the chicken legs for 3 to 5 minutes as needed to get a crisp crust, taking care not to burn them.

5. In a clean large bowl, mix the cheese and garlic oil.

6. Add the cooked chicken and toss well to coat.

7. Place coated chicken on the baking sheet and broil for an additional 5 to 6 minutes, rotating the chicken halfway through.

8. Take the chicken out of the oven and serve immediately.

Ingredient tip: Feel free to substitute chicken thighs or wings. In the case of wings, they make an excellent appetizer.

Per Serving: Calories: 398; Total Fat: 23g; Cholesterol: 157mg; Sodium: 527mg; Carbs: 1g; Sugar: 0g; Fiber: 0g; Protein: 47g

Bacon-Wrapped Chicken Livers with Ranch Dressing

Liver may sound like something your grandma used to eat, but its nutrient-dense profile is helping it make a comeback. These chicken livers can be eaten anytime—for breakfast, an afternoon or evening meal, or even a snack.

Serves 6

PREP TIME: **10 minutes**

COOK TIME: **20 minutes**

1 pound organic chicken livers, rinsed and patted dry

½ pound bacon, halved widthwise

Ranch Dressing (page 198), for dipping

1. Preheat the oven to broil. Place a baking rack on a rimmed baking sheet and line it with parchment paper.

2. Wrap each chicken liver in a piece of bacon and secure it with a toothpick. Place the wrapped livers on the prepared rack. Broil for 6 to 8 minutes. Turn them over and broil for 6 to 8 minutes on the other side.

3. Serve warm with ranch dressing for dipping.

Variation tip: If you don't tolerate the yogurt used in ranch dressing, make a honey-mustard dressing by mixing two parts pasteurized clover honey (2 tablespoons) with one part mustard (1 tablespoon). Taste and add more honey or mustard as desired.

Per Serving (with ¼ cup ranch dressing): Calories: 485; Total Fat: 40g; Cholesterol: 50mg; Sodium: 707mg; Carbs: 3g; Sugar: 0g; Fiber: 0g; Protein: 34g

Pesto Zoodles with Chicken

Zucchini has a high water content, so eating it can be a helpful way to stay hydrated. It's also high in vitamins A and C, potassium, and manganese.

Serves 4

PREP TIME: **10 minutes**

COOK TIME: **5 minutes**

1 tablespoon avocado oil

2 medium zucchini, peeled and spiralized into noodles (zoodles)

Salt

1 cup Zesty Arugula Pesto (page 200)

2 cups cubed and cooked organic chicken

⅓ cup freshly grated Parmesan cheese (optional)

1. Heat the avocado oil in a large skillet over medium-high heat.

2. Add the zoodles, sprinkle lightly with salt, and cook for about 4 minutes, or until tender, stirring frequently to cook evenly. Remove the pan from the heat and add the pesto. Mix thoroughly.

3. Divide the zoodles among four plates, top each with ½ cup of chicken, and sprinkle with Parmesan cheese (if using). Serve immediately.

Preparation tip: Zoodles can be made with a special spiralizer tool that can be purchased online or in local stores. You can also just peel the zucchini and use a vegetable peeler to make flat noodles.

Per Serving: Calories: 544; Total Fat: 47g; Cholesterol: 13mg; Sodium: 273mg; Carbs: 8g; Sugar: 3g; Fiber: 3g; Protein: 30g

Pressure Cooker
General Tso's Chicken

Once you make this chicken at home, your family will forget about Chinese takeout!

Serves 4

PREP TIME: **10 minutes**

COOK TIME: **20 minutes**

3 tablespoons arrowroot powder, plus 1 tablespoon if needed

1½ pounds skinless organic chicken thighs, cut into 2-inch pieces

2 tablespoons avocado oil

½ cup coconut aminos

⅓ cup white wine vinegar

2 tablespoons tomato paste

1 tablespoon pasteurized clover honey

1 tablespoon almond butter

¼ cup whole cane sugar, such as Sucanat, or granulated sugar

2 tablespoons peeled and chopped fresh ginger

1 tablespoon garlic oil

½ cup water

Cooked white rice, for serving (optional)

¼ cup chopped scallions, dark green parts only (optional)

1. In a large resealable plastic bag, combine 3 tablespoons of arrowroot powder and the chicken. Seal the bag and shake to coat the chicken.

2. On your pressure cooker, select Sauté and preheat the cooking pot.

3. Add the avocado oil.

4. Place the chicken in the pot and brown on each side. Select Cancel.

5. In a medium bowl, whisk the coconut aminos, vinegar, tomato paste, honey, almond butter, cane sugar, ginger, garlic oil, and water until fairly smooth. Pour the mixture over the chicken in the pressure cooker pot. Lock the lid in place and close the pressure release valve. Select the Manual function and cook on High Pressure for 8 minutes.

6. Do a Quick Release to vent the steam. Once completely vented, remove the lid. Check the sauce consistency. If it needs to be thicker, mix in another tablespoon of arrowroot powder, select Sauté, and cook for 5 minutes more. Serve the chicken immediately over white rice, if desired, topped with scallions (if using), or on its own.

Ingredient tip: Some stores sell precut chicken or smaller chicken tenders, which will reduce your prep time.

Per Serving: Calories: 664; Total Fat: 50g; Cholesterol: 30mg; Sodium: 845mg; Carbs: 30g; Sugar: 23g; Fiber: 1g; Protein: 23g

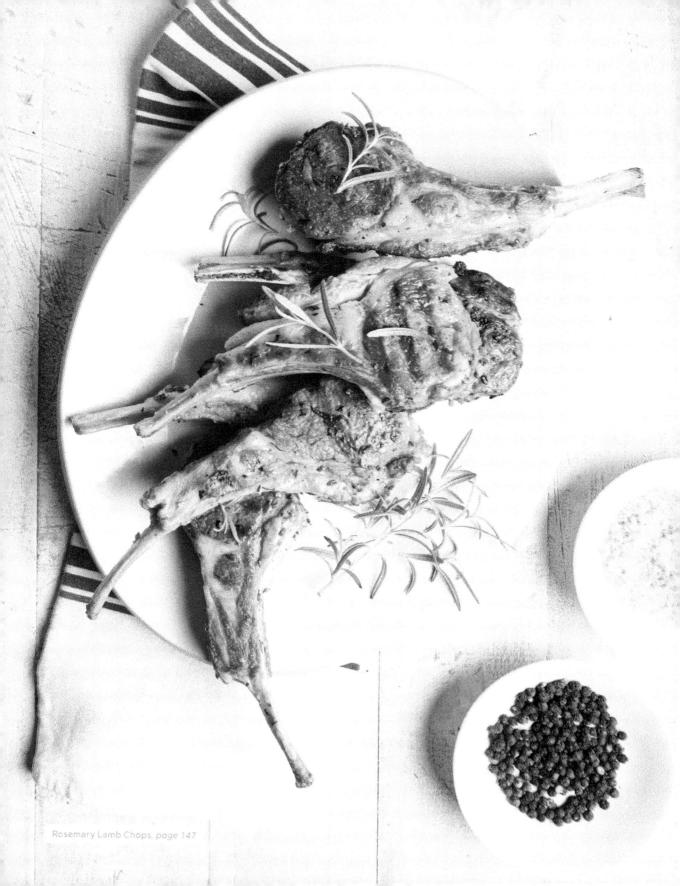

Rosemary Lamb Chops, page 147

Meat

Slow Cooker Roast Beef

Depending on your desired number of servings, you can use any size roast. If you use a much larger one than called for here, increase the other ingredients in proportion so you'll have enough gravy.

Serves 8

PREP TIME: **10 minutes**

COOK TIME: **9 hours**

2 cups Pressure Cooker Bone
Broth (page 92)

1 pound carrots, peeled and sliced,
or 1 pound baby carrots

2 tablespoons ghee, organic
grass-fed butter, or coconut oil

1 (3-pound) grass-fed chuck
roast or rump roast

Salt

1. In a slow cooker, combine the bone broth and carrots. Turn the cooker to low heat.

2. Heat a large skillet over high heat and melt the ghee in it.

3. Pat the roast dry with paper towels and generously season with salt. Place the roast in the skillet and sear for about 2 minutes on each side. Transfer the roast to the slow cooker, placing it on top of the carrots. Cover and cook for 9 hours on low heat.

4. Transfer the roast to a cutting board and cut into slices or chunks.

5. Using an immersion blender, or working in batches in a standard blender, blend the carrots, bone broth, and juices together to make a smooth gravy. Season to taste with salt.

6. Serve the roast topped with the gravy.

Make-ahead tip: This is an easy roast to cook overnight or start in the morning before work so you can come home to an almost-ready dinner.

Per Serving (made with ghee): Calories: 447; Total Fat: 23g; Cholesterol: 171mg; Sodium: 273mg; Carbs: 7g; Sugar: 4g; Fiber: 2g; Protein: 58g

Simple Steak

This steak is an easy weeknight meal but feels extra special. Use the best-quality meat you can afford.

Serves 4
PREP TIME: **5 minutes**
COOK TIME: **30 minutes**

1½ pounds grass-fed boneless sirloin, rib eye, or similar steak

Salt

Freshly ground black pepper (optional)

3 tablespoons ghee or coconut oil, divided

1. Pat the steak dry with paper towels and generously season both sides with salt and pepper (if using).

2. Heat a large skillet or cast-iron pan over high heat and melt 1 tablespoon of ghee in it.

3. Add the steak. Cook for 2 minutes. Flip the steak and add the remaining 2 tablespoons of ghee to the skillet. For the next 2 minutes, continuously baste the steak with the ghee by slightly tilting the pan to spoon up the ghee and pour it over the steak.

4. Flip, baste, and cook for 6 minutes more for medium-rare or 8 minutes for medium to medium-well. Transfer the steak to a cutting board. Cover loosely with aluminum foil and let rest for 10 minutes.

5. Cut the steak against the grain and divide it among four plates. Top with the ghee from the skillet. Serve immediately.

Ingredient tip: Buying grass-fed meat in bulk from a co-op or directly from the rancher allows you to get better-quality meat at a lower cost. CrowdCow.com is a service that works directly with ranchers.

Per Serving (made with sirloin): Calories: 311; Total Fat: 17g; Cholesterol: 0mg; Sodium: 90mg; Carbs: 0g; Sugar: 0g; Fiber: 0g; Protein: 39g

Pork Chops with Chimichurri Sauce

These oven-baked pork chops are elevated by the chimichurri sauce, but they're also delicious on their own or with a different sauce of your choosing. If you're following the Calming Menu, skip the chimichurri.

Serves 2

PREP TIME: **5 minutes**

COOK TIME: **25 minutes**

2 (5-ounce) thick-cut, bone-in pork chops

4 teaspoons melted ghee or avocado oil

Salt

Freshly ground black pepper

4 tablespoons Chimichurri Sauce (page 195), for serving

1. Preheat the oven to 400°F.

2. Heat an oven-safe skillet over high heat.

3. Pat the pork chops dry with paper towels, rub each one with 2 teaspoons of ghee, and generously sprinkle with salt and pepper. Place the pork chops in the pan and sear for 2 minutes on each side. Immediately transfer the skillet to the oven and cook for about 15 minutes, or until cooked through.

4. Let the chops rest for 5 minutes.

5. Top each chop with 2 tablespoons of chimichurri sauce and serve immediately.

Ingredient tip: This recipe also works with boneless pork chops or pork tenderloin. Cooking times may vary depending on your cut and size of meat.

Per Serving (made with ghee): Calories: 361; Total Fat: 0g; Cholesterol: 98mg; Sodium: 93mg; Carbs: 0g; Sugar: 0g; Fiber: 0g; Protein: 40g

Rosemary Lamb Chops

The word "natural" on a label is just a marketing term that can be used indiscriminately. Look for meat that is organic and 100 percent grass-fed. The best option for purchasing is to be part of a meat CSA (community-supported agriculture), or buy meat at a local co-op or farmers' market.

Serves 4

PREP TIME: **20 minutes**

COOK TIME: **10 minutes**

1 tablespoon sea salt

1 tablespoon finely chopped fresh rosemary (optional)

2 tablespoons garlic oil

8 grass-fed organic baby lamb chops

1 tablespoon beef tallow, pork fat, or ghee

1. In a small bowl, combine the salt, rosemary (if using), and garlic oil. Coat each lamb chop with this mixture and let the chops sit at room temperature for 15 minutes.

2. Heat a large skillet over high heat and melt the fat in it.

3. Add the lamb chops. Cook for 4 or 5 minutes on each side for medium-rare to medium. Serve immediately.

Ingredient tip: Rosemary is a beautifully fragrant herb that is easy to grow in a pot indoors, or outdoors in a pot or in the ground. You can snip off a sprig or two for a recipe or add it to a flower arrangement.

Per Serving (made with beef tallow): Calories: 313; Total Fat: 21g; Cholesterol: 99mg; Sodium: 1,740mg; Carbs: 0g; Sugar: 0g; Fiber: 0g; Protein: 29g

Pancetta-Wrapped Pork Tenderloin

Pork tenderloin is an easy weeknight meal that is made special with the addition of pancetta or bacon. The tenderloin is delicious on its own or can be eaten with a sauce of choice.

Serves 6

PREP TIME: **10 minutes**

COOK TIME: **40 minutes**

2 tablespoons chopped fresh rosemary

4 teaspoons herbes de Provence or dried Italian seasoning (without garlic)

2 teaspoons garlic oil

2 teaspoons extra-virgin olive oil

2 (1-pound) pork tenderloins

8 ounces pancetta, prosciutto, or bacon

Salt

Freshly ground black pepper

1. Preheat the oven to 350°F.

2. In a small bowl, stir together the rosemary, herbes de Provence, garlic oil, and olive oil. With clean hands or a pastry brush, spread the oil mixture over the tenderloins.

3. Wrap the pancetta around the oiled tenderloins and secure it by tying kitchen twine around the meat at 1- to 3-inch intervals as needed. Place the wrapped tenderloins on a rimmed baking sheet. Bake for 30 minutes.

4. Turn the oven to broil and broil for 5 minutes, or until the top is crispy.

5. Let the tenderloins rest for 10 minutes. Slice thinly, sprinkle with salt and pepper, and serve.

Ingredient tip: You can use pancetta, prosciutto, or bacon in this recipe, but they're all slightly different from one another. Both pancetta and bacon are cured meats made from the pork belly. Prosciutto is also cured but is made from the hind leg of a pig, called the ham.

Per Serving: Calories: 332; Total Fat: 18g; Cholesterol: 67mg; Sodium: 2,057mg; Carbs: 6g; Sugar: 2g; Fiber: 0g; Protein: 36g

Slow Cooker Pork and Pineapple

I adore using the slow cooker year-round. In summer, it means not having to use the oven and heat up the kitchen. In fall and winter, I love coming home to a warm, ready-made dish. I added a minimal amount of spices here, but if you tolerate them well, feel free to add more.

Serves 8

PREP TIME: **15 minutes**

COOK TIME: **8 hours**

Juice and zest of 2 organic oranges

Juice and zest of 2 organic limes

1 tablespoon garlic oil

1 teaspoon ground cumin

1 teaspoon chili powder (optional)

1 teaspoon dried oregano

1 teaspoon sea salt

½ teaspoon freshly ground black pepper

1 (2-pound) pork shoulder or butt roast

3 cups fresh pineapple chunks

1. Pour the orange juice and lime juice into the slow cooker.

2. In a small bowl, combine the orange zest, lime zest, garlic oil, cumin, chili powder (if using), oregano, salt, and pepper. Rub this mixture all over the pork, then place the pork in the slow cooker.

3. Sprinkle the pineapple chunks over the pork. Cook for 8 hours on low heat.

4. With two forks, shred the pork and mix it with the juices and pineapple.

Ingredient tip: Pineapple is an excellent source of vitamin C and manganese. One study showed that eating three or more servings of the fruit a day can protect against age-related macular degeneration, which can be associated with vision loss.

Per Serving (made with chili powder and pork shoulder):
Calories: 316; Total Fat: 19g; Cholesterol: 74mg; Sodium: 296mg; Carbs: 14g; Sugar: 12g; Fiber: 2g; Protein: 24g

Meat Loaf with Liver

If you're not a huge fan of the taste of liver but want to add it to your diet for its health benefits, meat loaf is your answer! This recipe is very basic, so feel free to try it as is or add chopped celery, carrots, or other vegetables you enjoy and tolerate.

Serves 8

PREP TIME: **15 minutes**

COOK TIME: **1 hour 30 minutes**

FOR THE GLAZE

3 tablespoons aged
   balsamic vinegar

2 tablespoons tomato paste

1 tablespoon apple cider vinegar

FOR THE MEAT LOAF

½ pound organic chicken livers

1 pound ground pork

1 pound grass-fed ground beef

2 large eggs

¼ cup chopped fresh chives or
   scallions, dark green parts only

2 tablespoons Italian seasoning
   (without garlic)

2 tablespoons coconut aminos

2 tablespoons apple cider vinegar

2 tablespoons garlic oil

1 teaspoon paprika (optional)

½ teaspoon sea salt

TO MAKE THE GLAZE

In a small bowl, whisk the balsamic vinegar, tomato paste, and cider vinegar until smooth. Set aside.

TO MAKE THE MEAT LOAF

1. Preheat the oven to 350°F. Line a baking sheet with aluminum foil.

2. In a food processor, purée the chicken livers. Transfer to a large bowl.

3. Add the pork, beef, eggs, chives, Italian seasoning, coconut aminos, vinegar, garlic oil, paprika (if using), and salt. With clean hands or a spoon, mix together all of the ingredients, making sure everything is evenly incorporated. Transfer to a loaf pan.

4. Spread the glaze over the top of the meat loaf. Place the loaf pan on the prepared sheet to catch any juices that may run over. Bake for 1 hour 30 minutes.

5. Remove from the oven and let sit for 5 to 10 minutes before serving.

Make-ahead tip: You can cut the loaf into slices and freeze individual pieces to take for lunches at a later point. You can also bake as individual muffins using silicone holders or a greased muffin tin.

Per Serving: Calories: 373; Total Fat: 24g; Cholesterol: 189mg; Sodium: 645mg; Carbs: 16g; Sugar: 5g; Fiber: 2g; Protein: 22g

Easy Flank Steak

Grass-fed beef contains more healthy omega-3 fats and vitamin E than conventionally raised beef. This flank steak recipe calls for an overnight marinade, and it's worth the tiny bit of extra effort!

Serves 4

PREP TIME: **10 minutes, plus overnight to marinate and 5 minutes to rest**

COOK TIME: **15 minutes**

2 tablespoons red wine vinegar or apple cider vinegar

1 teaspoon mustard (without garlic)

2 teaspoons pasteurized clover honey

2 tablespoons coconut aminos

½ teaspoon sea salt

¼ teaspoon smoked paprika (optional)

2 teaspoons chopped fresh rosemary

¼ cup extra-virgin olive oil

2 tablespoons garlic oil

1 to 2 pounds grass-fed flank steak

1. In a blender, combine the vinegar, mustard, honey, coconut aminos, salt, paprika, and rosemary. Blend until combined. Turn the blender to low and, while it's running, slowly add the olive oil and garlic oil. Blend until emulsified

2. Put the steak in a baking pan and pour the marinade over it, turning the meat to coat fully. Cover the pan and transfer to the refrigerator to let the steak marinate overnight.

3. Preheat a grill to high heat or place a grill pan over high heat.

4. Remove the steak from the marinade, scraping off any excess. Discard the marinade. Place the steak on the hot grill or grill pan and sear on both sides for about 1 minute total.

5. Reduce the heat to medium and cook for about 5 minutes per side, or until cooked to your desired doneness, taking care not to overcook the meat.

6. Let the steak rest for 5 minutes, then cut against the grain into thin strips and serve immediately.

Ingredient tip: Paprika is a nightshade, so if you have sensitivity to other nightshades, such as eggplant, potatoes, or tomatoes, omit it from this recipe.

Per Serving: Calories: 227; Total Fat: 9g; Cholesterol: 67mg; Sodium: 87mg; Carbs: 0g; Sugar: 0g; Fiber: 0g; Protein: 33g

Slow Cooker Beef Tacos

When you make these tacos, your family won't notice they're low-FODMAP. Set out the toppings so people can make their own. The meat can be eaten by itself or in a corn tortilla, on a salad, or as a lettuce wrap.

Serves 8

PREP TIME: **20 minutes**

COOK TIME: **8 to 10 hours**

1 (2-pound) grass-fed
    beef chuck roast

3 scallions, dark green
    parts only, chopped

¼ cup freshly squeezed lime juice

¼ cup organic tomato paste

2 tablespoons garlic oil

1½ tablespoons apple
    cider vinegar

2 teaspoons ground cumin

2 teaspoons sea salt

1 teaspoon dried oregano

¾ cup low-FODMAP beef bone
    broth or Pressure Cooker
    Bone Broth (page 92)

3 bay leaves

16 corn tortillas or lettuce
    leaves (optional)

½ cup fresh cilantro
    leaves, chopped

Toppings (optional): Fresh
    organic diced tomatoes, diced
    avocado, 1 cup shredded
    aged Cheddar cheese

1. Place the roast in a slow cooker.

2. In a small bowl, stir together the scallions, lime juice, tomato paste, garlic oil, vinegar, cumin, salt, oregano, and bone broth until combined. Add the bay leaves and pour the mixture over the roast. Cook for 8 to 10 hours on low heat.

3. Using two forks, shred the cooked meat in the slow cooker and mix it into the sauce.

4. Some people tolerate corn very well and some don't. If you haven't eaten corn in a while, start with a half tortilla to see how you tolerate it.

SIBO tip: Some people tolerate corn very well and some don't. If you haven't eaten corn in a while, start with half a tortilla to see how you tolerate it.

Per Serving: Calories: 220; Total Fat: 10g; Cholesterol: 0mg; Sodium: 539mg; Carbs: 22g; Sugar: 3g; Fiber: 3g; Protein: 11g

Slow Cooker Lamb Curry

If you don't tolerate or enjoy lamb, it's easy to substitute beef stew meat in this recipe. This curry can be served on its own or over rice.

Serves 8
PREP TIME: **15 minutes**
COOK TIME: **8 hours**

2 tablespoons coconut oil or ghee

3 pounds lamb stew meat

1 (14-ounce) can full-fat coconut milk (without gums)

1½ tablespoons peeled and grated fresh ginger

1 tablespoon garlic oil

1 tablespoon paprika (optional)

2 teaspoons ground coriander

2 teaspoons ground cumin

1 teaspoon ground turmeric

1 (14-ounce) can diced organic tomatoes, undrained

1½ teaspoons sea salt, or to taste

1. Heat a large skillet over high heat and melt the coconut oil in it.

2. Working in batches as needed, place the stew meat in the pan and brown the outside. Transfer each batch to the slow cooker after it's browned. Repeat until all of the meat is browned.

3. Add the coconut milk, ginger, garlic oil, paprika, coriander, cumin, turmeric, and tomatoes to the cooker. Mix the ingredients together to coat the meat. Set the slow cooker to low and cook for 8 hours, or until the lamb is tender.

4. Stir in the salt and serve immediately.

Ingredient tip: Lamb is an excellent source of protein, iron, zinc, selenium, and vitamin B12.

Per Serving (made with coconut oil): Calories: 371; Total Fat: 23g; Cholesterol: 110mg; Sodium: 575mg; Carbs: 5g; Sugar: 2g; Fiber: 2g; Protein: 36g

Beef Burrito Bowls

Make beef burrito bowls in advance for the week and have them ready for lunch or a quick dinner.

Serves 4

PREP TIME: **15 minutes**

COOK TIME: **15 minutes**

1 tablespoon garlic oil

1 small organic green bell pepper, diced

2 scallions, dark green parts only, sliced

1 pound grass-fed ground beef

1 teaspoon ground cumin

1 teaspoon paprika (optional)

1 teaspoon dried oregano

4 cups cooked white rice

1 cup shredded aged Cheddar cheese (optional)

1½ cups diced organic tomato

½ avocado, diced

2 tablespoons chopped fresh cilantro leaves

4 lime wedges

1. Heat the garlic oil in a large saucepan over medium-high heat.

2. Add the bell pepper. Sauté for 3 minutes.

3. Add the scallions. Sauté for 1 minute more.

4. Add the ground beef, cumin, paprika, and oregano. Cook for about 8 minutes, or until the meat is cooked through.

5. Divide the rice among four bowls. Top each with some of the ground beef mixture, Cheddar cheese (if using), diced tomato, avocado, cilantro, and a lime wedge. Serve immediately or keep refrigerated.

Ingredient tip: Once you get used to making these bowls in advance for lunch or dinner, start playing with different ingredient options. For instance, a base of mashed potatoes topped with ground turkey, vegetables, and Chimichurri Sauce (page 195) would be delicious.

Per Serving: Calories: 578; Total Fat: 24g; Cholesterol: 98mg; Sodium: 365mg; Carbs: 56g; Sugar: 4g; Fiber: 4g; Protein: 33g

Asian Ground Pork in Lettuce Cups

This dish requires a bit of prep time to chop the ingredients, but it's worth it because it takes ground pork to a whole new level. It can be served as an appetizer or a main meal.

Serves 4

PREP TIME: **20 minutes**

COOK TIME: **20 minutes**

1 pound ground pork

2 tablespoons garlic oil

2 carrots, finely chopped

2 teaspoons Chinese five-spice powder

4 scallions, dark green parts only, chopped

2 teaspoons gluten-free fish sauce (preferably Red Boat brand)

½ cup fresh cilantro leaves, chopped

½ cup fresh Thai basil leaves, chopped

⅓ cup fresh mint leaves, chopped

1 large or 2 small heads butter lettuce, leaves separated

½ English cucumber, peeled, seeded, and diced

1 pint organic cherry tomatoes, halved

1. Heat a large skillet over high heat, place the pork in it, and sauté for 5 to 7 minutes, or until almost cooked through.

2. Add the garlic oil, carrots, five-spice powder, and scallions. Cook for 5 to 10 minutes, or until the pork is completely cooked through and no pink remains. Remove from the heat and transfer to a large serving bowl. Allow the mixture to cool slightly.

3. Stir in the fish sauce, cilantro, basil, and mint.

4. Serve spoonfuls of the mixture in the lettuce leaves, topped with cucumber and tomatoes.

Ingredient tip: Chinese five-spice powder is typically a mixture of fennel, cinnamon, star anise, Szechuan pepper, and cloves. It is said to encompass the flavors of sweet, sour, bitter, pungent, and salty.

Per Serving: Calories: 155; Total Fat: 11g; Cholesterol: 4mg; Sodium: 410mg; Carbs: 13g; Sugar: 5g; Fiber: 3g; Protein: 4g

Spanish Short Ribs

These ribs are a special treat and are delicious over mashed potatoes, rice, or all by themselves.

Serves 4 to 6
PREP TIME: **15 minutes**
COOK TIME: **3 hours**
30 minutes

5 pounds beef short ribs

Salt

Freshly ground black pepper

3 tablespoons avocado oil

3 scallions, dark green parts only, coarsely chopped

2 celery stalks, coarsely chopped

1 carrot, coarsely chopped

1 cup dry red wine

1 tablespoon garlic oil

1 (14-ounce) can chopped organic tomatoes, with liquid (without garlic)

¼ cup organic tomato paste

1 fresh thyme sprig

6 cups Pressure Cooker Bone Broth (page 92)

1 cup dry sherry

Zest of 1 organic orange

½ ounce unsweetened chocolate, chopped

1 tablespoon unsalted organic grass-fed butter

2 teaspoons fresh thyme leaves

1. Preheat the oven to 300°F.

2. Pat the short ribs dry with paper towels and generously sprinkle with salt and pepper.

3. Heat the avocado oil in a Dutch oven over medium-high heat.

4. When the oil is hot but not smoking, add the ribs. Brown well on all sides for about 5 minutes. Remove them from the pan and set aside.

5. Add the scallions, celery, and carrot to the pan. Sauté for 5 minutes, stirring often, until the vegetables begin to caramelize.

6. Increase the heat to high. Add the red wine and boil until it is reduced by half, stirring as needed.

7. Add the garlic oil, tomatoes with their liquid, tomato paste, and thyme sprig and stir to combine.

8. Return the ribs and any accumulated liquid to the pan. Add the bone broth. Bring to a boil and transfer the pan to the oven. Bake, uncovered, for about 3 hours, until the meat is very tender. Remove the pan from the oven and transfer the ribs to a plate

9. Carefully strain the pan liquid into a large saucepan and stir in the sherry. Bring to a boil over medium-high heat and cook for 8 to 10 minutes, or until the liquid is reduced by one-third.

10. Add the orange zest, chocolate, butter, and thyme. Simmer, stirring, until the chocolate melts.

11. Add the ribs to the sauce in the pan and simmer for 5 minutes. Serve immediately.

Make-ahead tip: Individual portions can be frozen and reheated for lunch or dinner.

Per Serving: Calories: 1,073; Total Fat: 41g; Cholesterol: 5mg; Sodium: 397mg; Carbs: 29g; Sugar: 2g; Fiber: 2g; Protein: 134g

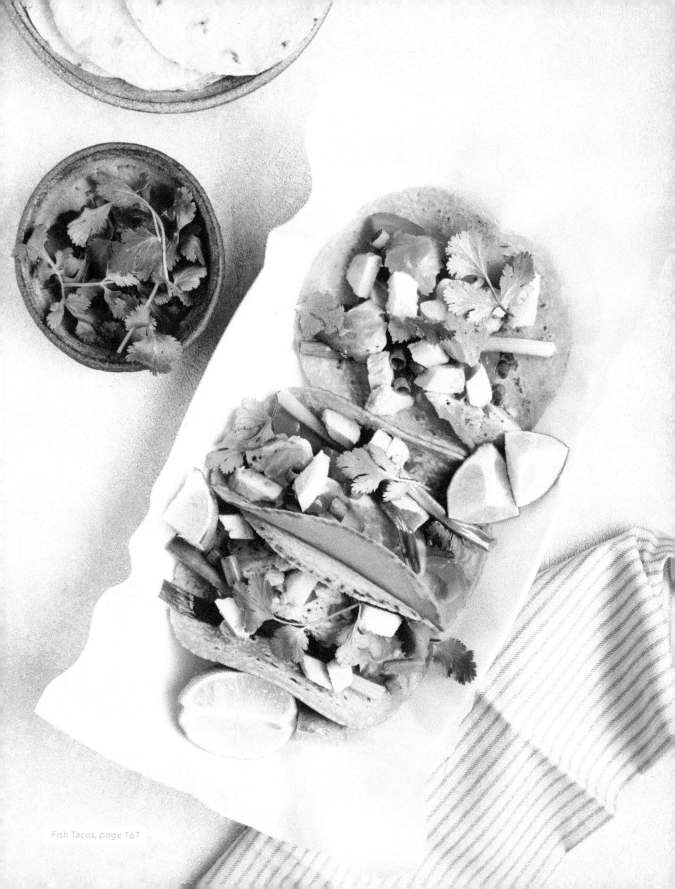

Fish Tacos, page 167

Fish and Seafood

12

Easy Baked White Fish

Sole and other flat fish are relatively low in calories and fat. Because we need healthy fat in our diet, we add olive oil here for extra taste and health benefits.

Serves 4
PREP TIME: **40 minutes**
COOK TIME: **20 minutes**

2 to 3 pounds cod or sole
Salt
¼ cup extra-virgin olive oil
4 lemon wedges
1 teaspoon chopped fresh parsley

1. Rinse the fish, pat dry with paper towels, and place in a baking pan.

2. Sprinkle with salt and the olive oil. Let marinate in the refrigerator for 30 minutes.

3. Preheat the oven to 350°F.

4. Bake the fish for 15 to 20 minutes, or until it is tender and flakes easily with a fork.

5. Squeeze the lemon wedges over the fish and sprinkle with the parsley. Serve immediately.

Make-ahead tip: Nobody wants to be the person microwaving leftover fish at the office, so it's best to make a portion you can eat at home within a day or two.

Per Serving: Calories: 309; Total Fat: 15g; Cholesterol: 133mg; Sodium: 854mg; Carbs: 1g; Sugar: 0g; Fiber: 0g; Protein: 43g

Tomato-Garlic Shrimp

This is an ideal recipe to make in the summer, when fragrant basil and juicy tomatoes are at their peak.

Serves 4
PREP TIME: **25 minutes**
COOK TIME: **5 minutes**

¼ cup extra-virgin olive oil

¼ cup garlic oil

Zest and juice of 1 lemon

1 tablespoon Dijon mustard (without garlic)

⅓ cup fresh parsley leaves, chopped, divided

¼ cup fresh basil leaves, chopped

2 tablespoons chopped chives

1 pint organic cherry tomatoes, halved

1 pound shrimp, peeled and deveined

Salt

Freshly ground black pepper

1. In a large bowl, combine the olive oil, garlic oil, lemon zest, lemon juice, mustard, ¼ cup of parsley, the basil, and chives. Mix thoroughly.

2. Add the tomatoes and shrimp. Stir to coat. Transfer the bowl to the refrigerator to let the shrimp marinate for 15 minutes.

3. Heat a large skillet over medium-high heat until hot.

4. Add the shrimp mixture. Sauté for about 5 minutes, or until the shrimp are cooked through, turning from translucent to pink and white.

5. Top with the remaining 1 tablespoon of parsley and serve immediately.

Ingredient tip: Cherry tomatoes are on the Dirty Dozen list (see page 204), so purchase organic whenever you can. If you do well with raw vegetables, they make an easily portable and delicious snack.

Per Serving: Calories: 340; Total Fat: 29g; Cholesterol: 165mg; Sodium: 643mg; Carbs: 6g; Sugar: 0g; Fiber: 2g; Protein: 16g

Honey-Mustard Salmon

Costco sells frozen wild-caught salmon for a reasonable price. Thaw individual pieces overnight in the refrigerator, and they will be ready to cook when you come home the next evening.

Serves 2

PREP TIME: **10 minutes**

COOK TIME: **18 minutes**

2 tablespoons mustard
(without garlic)

2 tablespoons pasteurized
clover honey

1 teaspoon freshly squeezed
lemon juice

1 teaspoon avocado oil

2 (5-ounce) salmon fillets

Salt

Freshly ground black pepper

1. Preheat the oven to 375°F. Line a rimmed baking sheet with aluminum foil.

2. In a small bowl, whisk the mustard, honey, and lemon juice until combined.

3. Spread the avocado oil in the middle of the piece of foil. Place the salmon fillets next to each other on top of the avocado oil. Generously season the fillets with salt and pepper.

4. Pour the honey-mustard sauce over the fish. Bring the sides of the aluminum foil together to form a sealed packet covering the salmon. Bake for 15 minutes.

5. Carefully open the foil packet to avoid any steam, exposing the salmon.

6. Turn the oven to broil and broil the fish for 3 minutes.

7. Using a spatula, transfer each piece of salmon to a dinner plate and serve immediately.

Ingredient tip: Salmon contains DHA and EPA, omega-3 fatty acids. These fats play a role in mood regulation, brain function, and decreasing inflammation.

Per Serving: Calories: 229; Total Fat: 5g; Cholesterol: 81mg; Sodium: 394mg; Carbs: 20g; Sugar: 17g; Fiber: 0g; Protein: 29g

Mahi-Mahi with Avocado-Lime Butter

The avocado-lime butter makes this dish special enough for a dinner party without extensive ingredients or extra time in the kitchen. The butter also tastes great on chicken or steak.

Serves 4

PREP TIME: **10 minutes**

COOK TIME: **10 minutes**

¼ cup salted ghee, organic grass-fed butter, or coconut oil, melted

2 tablespoons minced fresh cilantro leaves

½ small ripe avocado

1 tablespoon freshly squeezed lime juice

4 mahi-mahi fillets

Salt

Freshly ground black pepper

Paprika, for seasoning (optional)

1 tablespoon coconut oil or ghee

1. In a food processor or blender, combine the ghee, cilantro, avocado, and lime juice. Process until smooth. Transfer to a small bowl and set aside.

2. Pat the fish fillets dry with paper towels and generously sprinkle with salt, pepper, and paprika (if using).

3. Heat a skillet over medium-high heat and melt the coconut oil in it until it just begins to sizzle but not smoke.

4. Add the fillets to the skillet. Cook for 4 to 5 minutes per side, or until cooked through.

5. Divide the fish among four plates and top each fillet with one-quarter of the avocado-lime butter. Serve.

Ingredient tip: Making different flavored butters to top cooked meats and seafood not only adds healthy fats to your diet but also gives your food extra flavor. Try combining room temperature ghee or butter with garlic oil and fresh herbs, then roll into a log in plastic wrap. Keep refrigerated and cut off a slice to top your meat or seafood.

Per Serving: Calories: 267; Total Fat: 20g; Cholesterol: 115mg; Sodium: 101mg; Carbs: 1g; Sugar: 0g; Fiber: 1g; Protein: 21g

Lemon-Caper Salmon

Capers are commonly used in Mediterranean cuisines and are rich in rutin and quercetin, two flavonoids that are sources of antioxidants.

Serves 4
PREP TIME: **5 minutes**
COOK TIME: **10 minutes**

4 (5-ounce) salmon fillets

Salt

Freshly ground black pepper

1 tablespoon avocado oil

4 tablespoons ghee, organic grass-fed butter, or coconut oil

2 tablespoons freshly squeezed lemon juice

¼ cup capers, rinsed and drained

2 tablespoons chopped fresh parsley

1. Pat the salmon dry with paper towels and generously season with salt and pepper.

2. Heat a skillet over high heat and melt the avocado oil in it until hot but not smoking.

3. Add the salmon and cook for about 4 minutes per side, or until cooked through. Transfer the fillets to individual plates and set aside.

4. Return the skillet to medium-high heat and add the ghee, lemon juice, and capers. Cook for 1 minute, stirring, until the ghee is melted. Spoon the lemon-caper butter over each salmon fillet. Sprinkle the parsley on top and serve immediately.

Ingredient tip: Parsley shouldn't be relegated to just a decorative sprig on the side of the plate—it is an excellent source of folate, iron, and vitamins A, C, and K.

Per Serving: Calories: 453; Total Fat: 31g; Cholesterol: 0mg; Sodium: 381mg; Carbs: 1g; Sugar: 0g; Fiber: 0g; Protein: 39g

Ginger-Lime Swordfish Skewers

If it's summer, fire up the grill and include these in your next barbecue. In the winter, you can use a grill pan indoors.

Serves 4

PREP TIME: **2 hours**

COOK TIME: **10 minutes**

3 tablespoons freshly squeezed lime juice

3 tablespoons gluten-free fish sauce (preferably Red Boat brand; see Tip below)

3 tablespoons pasteurized clover honey

1 tablespoon peeled and chopped fresh ginger

1 tablespoon garlic oil

2 scallions, dark green parts only, chopped

1½ pounds swordfish fillets, cut into chunks

2 tablespoons avocado oil, divided

2 small organic red bell peppers, seeded and cut into large chunks

1. In a blender, combine the lime juice, fish sauce, honey, ginger, garlic oil, and scallions. Blend until puréed.

2. Place the swordfish on a baking pan and pour the marinade over it, making sure the fish is fully coated. Cover and refrigerate for 1½ hours.

3. Preheat a grill to high or place a grill pan over high heat.

4. Brush 8 metal skewers, or 8 wooden skewers soaked in water, with half of the avocado oil. Remove the fish from the refrigerator and wipe away any excess marinade. Discard the marinade. Thread the swordfish onto the skewers, alternating with the bell pepper chunks. Lightly brush the finished skewers with the remaining avocado oil.

5. Grill the skewers for about 4 minutes per side, or until cooked through. Serve immediately.

Ingredient tip: Red Boat brand fish sauce is minimally processed and only made from fresh-caught wild black anchovies and sea salt.

Per Serving: Calories: 436; Total Fat: 19g; Cholesterol: 84mg; Sodium: 1,259mg; Carbs: 21g; Sugar: 18g; Fiber: 2g; Protein: 44g

Cod with Tomato-Basil Sauce

Cod is an excellent source of vitamin B$_{12}$, iodine, selenium, and phosphorus. This simple and quick recipe highlights the fresh fish.

Serves 4
PREP TIME: **15 minutes**
COOK TIME: **25 minutes**

2 tablespoons garlic oil

2 cups cherry tomatoes, halved

¼ cup low-FODMAP chicken broth (see Resources, page 206) or dry white wine

½ cup fresh basil leaves, chopped

Zest of 1 lemon

2 tablespoons freshly squeezed lemon juice

4 cod fillets

Salt

Freshly ground black pepper

2 tablespoons avocado oil, coconut oil, or ghee

1. Heat the garlic oil in a medium skillet over medium heat.

2. Add the tomatoes. Cook for 3 minutes.

3. Pour in the chicken broth and bring to a low boil.

4. Stir in the basil, lemon zest, and lemon juice. Reduce the heat to medium-low and simmer the sauce for 8 minutes.

5. Meanwhile, pat the fish dry with paper towels and generously sprinkle with salt and pepper.

6. In a separate medium or large skillet over medium-high heat, heat the avocado oil.

7. Place the cod in the skillet and cook for 4 to 5 minutes on each side, or until cooked through. Divide the fish among four plates and top with the tomato-basil sauce. Serve immediately.

Ingredient tip: This recipe is best made during the summer months when basil and tomatoes are at their peak.

Per Serving: Calories: 225; Total Fat: 0g; Cholesterol: 60mg; Sodium: 221mg; Carbs: 5g; Sugar: 2g; Fiber: 2g; Protein: 15g

Fish Tacos

Fish tacos are perfect for a casual weeknight dinner.

Serves 4
PREP TIME: **10 minutes**
COOK TIME: **15 minutes**

1 tablespoon coconut
   or avocado oil

4 scallions, dark green
   parts only, chopped

1 pound wild-caught salmon or
   other wild-caught fish fillets

2 cups diced organic tomatoes

⅓ cup fresh cilantro
   leaves, chopped

3 tablespoons freshly
   squeezed lime juice

1 tablespoon garlic oil

Salt

Freshly ground black pepper

8 small corn tortillas, warmed,
   or large butter lettuce or
   romaine lettuce leaves

½ avocado, cut into pieces

1. Heat a large skillet over high heat and melt the coconut oil in it.

2. Add the scallions. Cook for about 4 minutes, or until softened.

3. Place the salmon fillets in the pan. Cook for about 4 minutes per side, or until cooked through. Break the fillets into larger chunks and add the tomatoes, cilantro, and lime juice. Mix together and cook for 5 minutes. Remove from the heat, add the garlic oil, stir, and season to taste with salt and pepper.

4. Place 2 tortillas or lettuce leaves on each plate. Fill with the fish mixture and top with avocado pieces. Serve immediately.

Serving tip: This fish mixture can be eaten in corn tortillas, lettuce leaves, over rice, or on its own.

Per Serving (made with coconut oil and corn tortillas): Calories: 442; Total Fat: 26g; Cholesterol: 68mg; Sodium: 420mg; Carbs: 30g; Sugar: 6g; Fiber: 7g; Protein: 22g

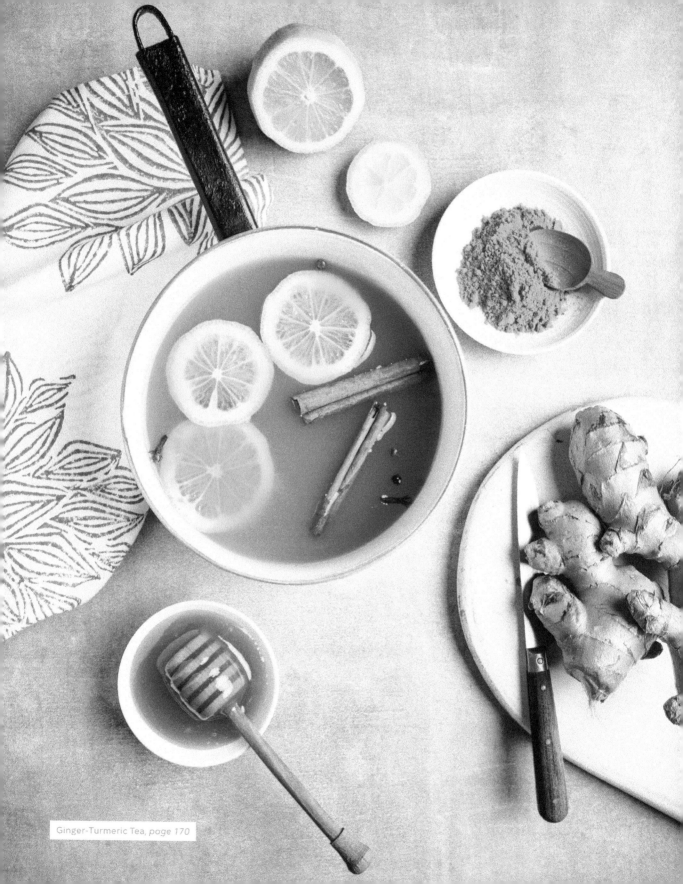

Ginger-Turmeric Tea, page 170

Drinks and Snacks

13

Ginger-Turmeric Tea

This soothing tea combines ginger, which is great for mitigating nausea, and turmeric, a powerful anti-inflammatory. Adding black pepper makes the turmeric more bioavailable. This tea can be enjoyed warm or cold.

Serves 4

PREP TIME: **10 minutes**

COOK TIME: **15 minutes**

4 cups cold water or weak black tea

1 (3-inch) piece fresh turmeric root, peeled and cut into large pieces

1 (3-inch) piece fresh ginger, peeled and cut into large pieces

¼ cup pasteurized clover honey or maple syrup

2 whole cloves (optional)

2 star anise (optional)

1 cinnamon stick (optional)

1 teaspoon peppercorns or freshly ground black pepper

½ large lemon, quartered

1. In a blender, combine the water, turmeric, and ginger. Blend on high speed until the turmeric and ginger are chopped. Transfer to a medium saucepan and place over high heat.

2. Add the honey, the cloves, star anise, and cinnamon stick (if using), and the peppercorns. Bring just to a boil. Reduce the heat to low and simmer for 10 minutes. Strain the mixture and discard the spices.

3. Pour into four mugs and garnish each with a lemon wedge.

Preparation tip: If you prefer a vegan tea, use maple syrup as your sweetener. This tea can be quite powerful, so feel free to dilute to your preference. Black pepper is in the nightshade family, so if you react to nightshades, omit it.

Per Serving: Calories: 76; Total Fat: 0g; Cholesterol: 0mg; Sodium: 8mg; Carbs: 20g; Sugar: 17g; Fiber: 1g; Protein: 0g

Sautéed Banana

This recipe is a simple, delicious snack or dessert when you want something sweet.

Serves 1
PREP TIME: **5 minutes**
COOK TIME: **5 minutes**

1 teaspoon to 1 tablespoon ghee, organic grass-fed butter, or coconut oil (see Ingredient tip)

1 teaspoon to 1 tablespoon pasteurized clover honey or maple syrup (see Ingredient tip)

1 firm, unripe medium banana, sliced

1. In a small saucepan over high heat, combine the ghee and honey and stir to melt.

2. When the ghee and honey begin to sizzle, add the sliced banana. Reduce the heat to medium-high and sauté for 1 to 2 minutes, or until the banana begins to soften (but you don't want it too mushy!) and the mixture begins to caramelize.

3. Remove from the heat, transfer the banana and sauce to a plate, and enjoy.

Ingredient tip: If you tolerate both honey and coconut oil, use a full tablespoon of both—it makes the banana saucier. You may also prefer a different ratio of honey to butter, depending on your sweet tooth.

SIBO tip: Unripe bananas contain resistant starch, which may cause symptoms in some people. If you tolerate banana, they are a great on-the-go snack food and are a helpful ingredient in many recipes.

Per Serving (made with ghee and honey): Calories: 154; Total Fat: 5g; Cholesterol: 0g; Sodium: 0mg; Carbs: 18g; Sugar: 12g; Fiber: 3g; Protein: 1g

Chicken Chips

When you're craving something crunchy and salty—chicken chips to the rescue! They are similar to pork rinds but taste so much better because they're fresh out of the oven.

Serves 3

PREP TIME: **5 minutes**

COOK TIME: **15 minutes**

6 organic chicken skins of similar size, from any parts

Salt

Freshly ground black pepper

Other spices as desired, such as curry, cumin, or chili powder, for seasoning

1. Preheat the oven to 425°F.

2. Pat the skins dry with paper towels and stretch them out on a rimmed baking sheet, making them as thin as possible. Depending on size, up to 6 skins will fit on one sheet.

3. Sprinkle with salt, pepper, and any other spices desired.

4. Bake for 12 to 15 minutes. If the skins don't look crispy, broil until they're crisp.

Ingredient tip: If you eat organic chicken skins from healthy animals, you consume fats your body needs to support healthy cells, skin, and brain function. Fat also helps our bodies use fat-soluble vitamins A, E, D, and K.

Per Serving: Calories: 259; Total Fat: 23g; Cholesterol: 47mg; Sodium: 86mg; Carbs: 0g; Sugar: 0g; Fiber: 0g; Protein: 12g

Sour Gummies

Gummies make a great snack and can give you a protein boost when you're on the go. They're also a fun snack for kids—you don't have to tell them they're healthy, too!

Makes about 25 gummies, depending on mold size

PREP TIME: **10 minutes, plus 15 to 30 minutes to set**

COOK TIME: **5 minutes**

1 cup freshly squeezed lemon juice or lime juice

3 tablespoons grass-fed gelatin powder (Great Lakes brand)

⅓ cup pasteurized clover honey

1 teaspoon vanilla extract (optional)

1. Put silicone molds onto a baking sheet. Alternatively, use an 8-by-8-inch glass pan.

2. Pour the lemon juice into a small saucepan and sprinkle the gelatin over it. Let the gelatin dissolve and add the honey and vanilla (if using).

3. Place the pan over low heat and whisk the ingredients to incorporate as they begin to melt, about 5 minutes.

4. Transfer the gummy mixture into a glass measuring cup or other container with a spout for easy pouring. Pour the gummy mixture into the molds. Let set for 15 to 30 minutes, or until solid.

5. Remove the gummies from the molds and keep refrigerated for 1 to 2 weeks.

Ingredient tip: If you don't like mouth-puckering sour flavors, substitute coconut or nut milk, or a fruit purée, like organic strawberry, for half the citrus juice.

Substitution tip: Another low-FODMAP milk, juice, or fruit purée can be substituted for the lemon juice.

Per Serving (1 gummy): Calories: 18; Total Fat: 0g; Cholesterol: 0mg; Sodium: 3mg; Carbs: 4g; Sugar: 4g; Fiber: 0g; Protein: 1g

Ginger Limeade

For those losing excessive weight or who are underweight, adding calories via drinks like this refreshing one can be a help.

Serves 6

PREP TIME: **5 minutes**

5 cups water, plus more as needed

1 cup Honey-Ginger Simple Syrup (page 194), plus more as needed

¾ cup freshly squeezed lime juice (from about 6 limes), plus more as needed

In a large pitcher, stir together the water, simple syrup, and lime juice. Taste and adjust with more water, simple syrup, and/or lime juice as desired.

Variation tip: This can also be made with lemon juice for a ginger lemonade. Alternatively, make the honey simple syrup without ginger for a regular lemonade.

Per Serving: Calories: 134; Total Fat: 0g; Cholesterol: 0g; Sodium: 12mg; Carbs: 35g; Sugar: 33g; Fiber: 0g; Protein: 0g

Satisfying Smoothie

A smoothie should incorporate healthy fats, protein, and carbohydrates in the form of low-FODMAP grains, fruits, or vegetables. This recipe gives you lots of options based on what's available and whatever sounds good. It can be used as a meal replacement or in addition to your meal if you need to add calories. If you're using a lot of ingredients, don't worry if the smoothie turns brown—it will still be delicious!

Serves 1

PREP TIME: **10 minutes**

1 tablespoon MCT oil, melted ghee, or coconut oil

1 tablespoon low-FODMAP nut butter or whole nuts (optional)

1 to 2 cups nut, coconut milk, or lactose-free milk, or water

1 to 2 tablespoons collagen hydrolysate (Great Lakes or Vital Proteins brands) or low-FODMAP protein powder (optional)

1 tablespoon pasteurized clover honey or maple syrup

¼ cup cooked white rice, quinoa, butternut squash, Kabocha squash, pumpkin, or sweet potato (optional)

1 cup fresh or frozen low-FODMAP fruits or vegetables of choice, including zucchini, spinach, blueberries, strawberries, kiwi, or banana

1 teaspoon to 1 tablespoon flavoring, such as ground cinnamon, ground cardamom, vanilla extract, or cocoa powder

Ice, as needed, for thickness

In a blender, combine all the ingredients as desired. Blend thoroughly. Add additional water or ice as needed.

Ingredient tip: Recommended flavor combinations include:

> Milk of choice + coconut oil + nut butter + banana + clover honey + cocoa

> Milk of choice + collagen hydrolysate + maple syrup + white rice + ground cinnamon + zucchini

> Milk of choice + collagen hydrolysate + spinach + frozen blueberries + clover honey

> For a vegan smoothie, use maple syrup as your sweetener and the MCT or coconut oil for your fat.

Per Serving (made with MCT oil, almond butter, almond milk, Great Lakes collagen hydrolysate, clover honey, white rice, spinach, and cinnamon): Calories: 451; Total Fat: 26g; Cholesterol: 0mg; Sodium: 308mg; Carbs: 39g; Sugar: 19g; Fiber: 6g; Protein: 23g

Blueberry-Coconut Milk

Homemade coconut milk tastes so much better than anything from the store! Adding blueberries makes this a great drink on its own or a wonderful addition to smoothies.

Serves 6

PREP TIME: **15 minutes, plus 30 minutes to sit**

1 cup organic unsweetened shredded coconut (preferably Let's Do . . . Organic brand)

1 cup blueberries, fresh or frozen and thawed

6 cups boiling water, plus more as needed

1 to 2 tablespoons pasteurized clover honey (optional, depending on your desired sweetness)

1 to 2 teaspoons vanilla extract (optional)

1. In a blender, combine the coconut and blueberries.

2. Pour in the boiling water until the blender is about three-fourths full.

3. Add the honey (if using). Let sit for 30 minutes, or until lukewarm.

4. Add the vanilla (if using). Blend on high speed for 1 minute. Transfer the mixture to a nut milk bag and strain the liquid into a bowl.

5. Squeeze any liquid out of the bag until the coconut is mostly dry. Discard the solids. Transfer the milk to a storage container. Keep refrigerated and consume within 3 to 4 days.

Variation tip: If you want regular coconut milk, omit the blueberries. You can also substitute other fruits, such as organic strawberries.

Per Serving (made with honey and vanilla): Calories: 124; Total Fat: 9g; Cholesterol: 0mg; Sodium: 10mg; Carbs: 8g; Sugar: 6g; Fiber: 4g; Protein: 1g

Homemade Electrolyte Drink

If you are an athlete or diarrhea is part of your symptom picture, replenishing with an electrolyte drink may make all the difference. Unfortunately, store-bought beverages are expensive and often contain excessive amounts of processed sugar and food coloring. This homemade version has healthy ingredients and is easy to make.

Serves 4

PREP TIME: **5 minutes**

3 cups tea (green, honeybush, rooibos, or peppermint) or water

1 cup coconut water

¼ cup freshly squeezed lemon juice or orange juice

2 tablespoons pasteurized clover honey or maple syrup

¼ teaspoon pink Himalayan salt or sea salt (such as Real Salt brand)

In a blender, combine the tea, coconut water, lemon juice, honey, and salt. Process until all of the honey dissolves. Transfer to a pitcher or individual Mason jars and keep refrigerated.

Preparation tip: If you prefer a vegan drink, use maple syrup as your sweetener.

Make-ahead tip: Make a double batch on the weekend and pour it into individual pint-size Mason jars to easily take with you.

Per Serving (made with green tea, lemon juice, and clover honey):
Calories: 48; Total Fat: 0g; Cholesterol: 0mg; Sodium: 264mg; Carbs: 14g; Sugar: 12g; Fiber: 0g; Protein: 0g

Mixed Nuts

Nuts can be hard to digest for many people. Make sure to chew them thoroughly and shoot for eating ⅓ cup or less at a time, unless you tolerate them very well.

Serves 12

PREP TIME: **5 minutes**

COOK TIME: **20 minutes**

4 cups raw almonds, macadamia nuts, walnuts, or pecans, or a combination

3 tablespoons maple syrup

2 tablespoons extra-virgin olive oil, coconut oil, organic grass-fed butter, or ghee

2 tablespoons fresh rosemary, thyme, or sage, or a combination

1 teaspoon smoked paprika (optional)

2 teaspoons sea salt, plus more as needed

Freshly ground black pepper

1. Preheat the oven to 350°F. Line a baking sheet with parchment paper.

2. On the prepared sheet, combine the nuts, maple syrup, olive oil, herbs, paprika (if using), and 2 teaspoons of salt. Season to taste with pepper. Mix to combine.

3. Bake for 15 to 20 minutes, stirring twice during the baking time, making sure the nuts are evenly distributed on the baking sheet.

4. Remove from the oven, stir, and set on a wire rack to cool.

5. Taste and season with additional salt or pepper as desired.

SIBO tip: These nuts are great to bring to a cocktail party when you want something to munch on but don't want to call extra attention to yourself for needing "special" food. You can also put them in half-pint Mason jars tied with a ribbon for a lovely hostess or holiday gift.

Per Serving (made with pecans, walnuts, almonds, extra-virgin olive oil, and rosemary): Calories: 365; Total Fat: 34g; Cholesterol: 0mg; Sodium: 393mg; Carbs: 12g; Sugar: 6g; Fiber: 4g; Protein: 8g

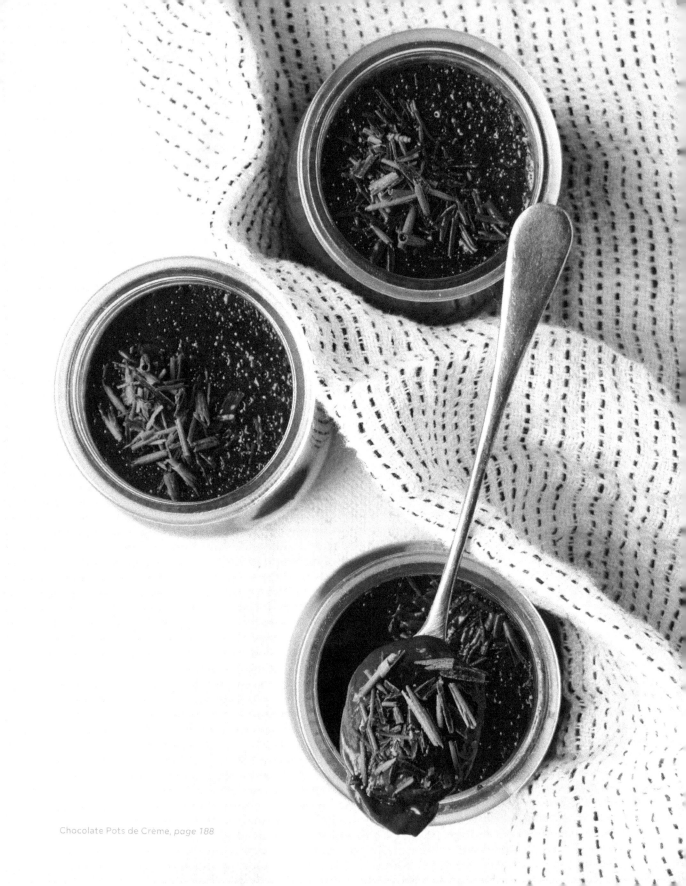

Chocolate Pots de Creme, page 188

Dessert

Lime Curd

Lime curd makes an excellent dessert by itself, or it can be used as a topping for pancakes or muffins.

Serves 4

PREP TIME: **10 minutes**

COOK TIME: **10 minutes**

3 large eggs

⅓ cup pasteurized clover honey

1 tablespoon lime zest

½ cup freshly squeezed lime juice

6 tablespoons ghee, organic grass-fed butter, or coconut oil

1. In a medium saucepan, whisk the eggs, honey, and lime zest until well mixed.

2. Add the lime juice and whisk to incorporate it.

3. Place the saucepan over medium heat and add the ghee. Continue to whisk while the fat melts. When the curd has thickened and a few bubbles pop on the surface, remove from the heat.

4. Set a fine-mesh sieve over a bowl and strain the mixture through it. Leave the curd in the bowl or transfer to four individual ramekins. Keep refrigerated for about 1 week.

Variation tip: Lemon or orange zest and juice can be substituted for lime in this delicious curd recipe.

Per Serving (made with ghee): Calories: 344; Total Fat: 26g; Cholesterol: 140mg; Sodium: 55mg; Carbs: 24g; Sugar: 22g; Fiber: 0g; Protein: 5g

Creamy Cardamom Custard

This custard makes a great breakfast, dessert, or snack because it's full of protein and healthy fat.

Serves 8
PREP TIME: **10 minutes, plus several hours to chill**
COOK TIME: **35 minutes**

8 large eggs

3 cups nut, coconut, or lactose-free milk

½ cup pasteurized clover honey or maple syrup (or less depending on your desired sweetness)

1 teaspoon vanilla extract

1 teaspoon ground cardamom

1. Preheat the oven to 350°F.

2. Bring a kettle of water (about 8 cups) to a boil.

3. In a blender, combine the eggs, milk, honey, vanilla, and cardamom. Process until well blended. Pour the custard into eight medium ramekins and place them in a roasting pan. Create a water bath by filling the roasting pan with boiling water so that it is about halfway up the sides of the ramekins. Bake for about 35 minutes (more or less time depending on your desired custard texture).

4. Wearing oven mitts, carefully remove the ramekins from the water bath. Let the water cool and discard it.

5. Let the individual custards chill in the refrigerator for several hours before serving.

Variation tip: If you don't like cardamom, leave it out and top the custards with a dusting of ground cinnamon or nutmeg as desired.

Per Serving (made with unsweetened coconut milk and clover honey): Calories: 149; Total Fat: 7g; Cholesterol: 185mg; Sodium: 72mg; Carbs: 18g; Sugar: 16g; Fiber: 1g; Protein: 6g

Vanilla-Orange Fat Bombs

Enjoy these fat bombs as a snack or toss some into a blender with a cup of hot coffee or tea. They'll make the beverage frothy and creamy while also adding healthy fat.

Yield varies depending on the size of the mold

PREP TIME: **5 minutes, plus 30 minutes to chill**

COOK TIME: **15 minutes**

1 cup coconut butter or manna

1 cup coconut milk (without gums)

Zest of 1 organic orange

2 tablespoons pasteurized clover honey

Juice of 2 organic oranges

1 tablespoon vanilla extract

1. In a small saucepan over low heat, combine the coconut butter, coconut milk, orange zest, and honey. Cook, stirring, until combined and warmed through.

2. Remove from the heat and stir in the orange juice and vanilla. Pour the mixture into silicone molds (like gummy molds) and refrigerate or freeze until firm, about 30 minutes.

3. Remove from the molds and store in the freezer.

Ingredient tip: Food-grade cocoa butter can be substituted for the coconut manna as desired and gives it a very slight chocolate taste.

Per Serving (2 fat bombs): Calories: 140; Total Fat: 14g; Cholesterol: 0mg; Sodium: 77mg; Carbs: 4g; Sugar: 3g; Fiber: 0g; Protein: 0g

Roasted Orange Rhubarb

This rhubarb can be enjoyed on its own, over rice cereal for breakfast, or topped with lactose-free cream or coconut cream.

Serves 4
PREP TIME: **10 minutes**
COOK TIME: **20 minutes**

1 cup dry vermouth

¼ cup pasteurized clover honey or whole cane sugar, such as Sucanat

2 tablespoons freshly squeezed orange juice

Zest of ½ organic orange

8 rhubarb stalks, edges trimmed

1. Preheat the oven to 350°F.

2. In a small bowl, whisk the vermouth, honey, orange juice, and orange zest until combined.

3. Place the rhubarb stalks in a baking dish and top with the vermouth mixture. Cover the baking dish with aluminum foil or a lid. Bake for about 20 minutes, or until the rhubarb softens and is very tender.

Preparation tip: If you prefer a vegan dish, use the cane sugar.

Ingredient tip: Rhubarb is typically considered a vegetable, but in North America is mostly used as a fruit in sweet dishes.

Per Serving (made with clover honey): Calories: 116; Total Fat: 0g; Cholesterol: 0mg; Sodium: 162mg; Carbs: 24g; Sugar: 20g; Fiber: 3g; Protein: 44g

Nut Butter Cupcakes with Cream Cheese Frosting

You can buy lactose-free cream cheese or add lactase drops (see Resources, page 206) to regular cream cheese. These are perfectly festive for a birthday party and taste even better than traditional cupcakes.

Makes about 16 cupcakes
PREP TIME: **10 minutes**
COOK TIME: **45 minutes**

FOR THE CUPCAKES

2 cups almond butter
   or pecan butter

1 cup pasteurized clover honey

½ teaspoon baking soda

4 large eggs

FOR THE FROSTING

2 (8-ounce) packages lactose-
   free cream cheese

½ cup pasteurized clover honey

1 tablespoon vanilla extract

TO MAKE THE CUPCAKES

1. Preheat the oven to 300°F.

2. In a medium bowl, combine the nut butter, honey, baking soda, and eggs. Stir to combine. Evenly divide the batter among 16 silicone baking cups or two oiled and lined 8-cup cupcake pans (for 16 cupcakes). Bake for about 32 minutes, or until a cupcake springs back when lightly touched.

TO MAKE THE FROSTING

In the bowl of a stand mixer or in a medium bowl using an immersion blender or handheld electric mixer, whip the cream cheese, honey, and vanilla. Set aside.

1. When the cupcakes are done, transfer them to a wire rack to cool for 10 minutes. Remove the cupcakes from the pan and let them cool completely. When cool, remove the cupcakes from their silicone liners, if used.

2. Frost with the cream cheese frosting. Serve immediately or refrigerate until ready to serve.

Ingredient tip: If you don't tolerate dairy, these cupcakes taste great with a variety of other frostings, including ones that are coconut- or chocolate-based.

Per Serving (1 cupcake): Calories: 426; Total Fat: 30g; Cholesterol: 80mg; Sodium: 125mg; Carbs: 33g; Sugar: 26g; Fiber: 4g; Protein: 10g

Chocolate Pots de Crème

This dessert is perfect to serve at a dinner party or make for yourself.

Serves 6

PREP TIME: **15 minutes, plus 2 hours to chill**

COOK TIME: **40 minutes**

6 large egg yolks

¼ cup pasteurized clover honey

1½ cups full-fat coconut milk or lactose-free half-and-half

6 ounces dairy-free dark chocolate (70% cacao or higher)

3 tablespoons whiskey (optional)

Coconut milk whipped cream or lactose-free whipped cream, for serving (optional)

1. Preheat the oven to 350°F.

2. Place six ramekins in a roasting pan. Bring a kettle of water (about 8 cups) to a boil.

3. In a large bowl, whisk the egg yolks and honey for about 3 minutes until well combined. Set aside.

4. In a medium or large saucepan over medium-high heat, bring the coconut milk to a simmer, stirring occasionally. Remove from the heat and add the chocolate, whisking until it's melted. Pour the chocolate mixture over the egg yolks and honey, whisking well to combine.

5. Add the whiskey (if using) and whisk to incorporate. Divide the mixture evenly among the ramekins. Create a water bath by filling the roasting pan with boiling water so that it is about halfway up the sides of the ramekins.

6. Carefully transfer the pan to the oven and bake for 30 to 40 minutes, or until the pots de crème appear set. Carefully remove the pan from the oven. Transfer the ramekins to the refrigerator to chill for at least 2 hours, or until ready to serve.

7. If desired, top with whipped cream and serve.

Variation tip: Substitute 3 tablespoons of brewed espresso for the whiskey; it deepens the chocolate taste—just make sure not to eat it too late in the day if you're very sensitive to caffeine.

Per Serving (made with whiskey): Calories: 276; Total Fat: 23g; Cholesterol: 185mg; Sodium: 18mg; Carbs: 18g; Sugar: 18g; Fiber: 0g; Protein: 4g

Peppermint Marshmallows

These are a delicious treat for young and old and can make a fun family activity. Be extra careful when pouring the hot mixture into the stand mixer.

Makes 20 marshmallows
PREP TIME: **5 minutes**
COOK TIME: **20 minutes**

1 tablespoon organic grass-fed butter, ghee, or coconut oil

1 cup water, divided

3 tablespoons grass-fed gelatin powder (such as Great Lakes brand)

1 cup pasteurized clover honey

¼ teaspoon sea salt

1 teaspoon peppermint extract

Crushed nuts, powdered sugar, shredded coconut, or almond flour, for coating (optional)

1. Grease an 8-by-8-inch pan with the butter and line it with parchment paper in both directions, with a little parchment hanging over all four sides.

2. Put ½ cup of water in the bowl of a stand mixer and sprinkle the gelatin over it.

3. In a medium saucepan over medium-high heat, combine the remaining ½ cup of water, the honey, and salt. Clip a candy thermometer to the pan. Bring the mixture to a boil, then let boil for about 8 minutes, or until it reaches 240°F. Immediately remove the pan from the heat.

4. Turn the mixer to medium-low speed and slowly and carefully pour the hot honey mixture into the bowl.

5. Mix in the peppermint extract.

6. Once the mixture is combined, turn the mixer to high speed and continue to beat until the mixture turns white and is thickened, like marshmallow crème, about 5 minutes.

7. Turn off the mixer and immediately scrape the marshmallow into the prepared pan, smoothing the top.

> **CONTINUED**

8. Add the optional coatings as desired to cover the top of the marshmallows. Remove the marshmallows from the pan by pulling on the flaps of the parchment and turn the marshmallows out onto a cutting board. Remove the parchment and sprinkle the coating (if using) on the uncovered side of the marshmallows. Cut the marshmallows into 20 squares and roll in additional coating, if desired. Store in a glass container. Eat individually or use in hot chocolate.

SIBO tip: These marshmallows aren't introduced until Week 4 because they have a higher level of sugar (in the form of honey), and many people with SIBO do better with smaller amounts of sugar. If you tolerate sugar well and are missing sweets, try this recipe sooner.

Per Serving (2 marshmallows, made with butter and no toppings):
Calories: 114; Total Fat: 1g; Cholesterol: 3mg; Sodium: 58mg; Carbs: 26g; Sugar: 26g; Fiber: 0g; Protein: 2g

Chocolate-Pecan Nut Butter

Homemade nut butter is easy to make and tastes so much better than what you get from the store.

Makes about 2 cups

PREP TIME: **5 minutes**

COOK TIME: **25 minutes**

1 pound raw pecans

1 teaspoon sea salt, plus more as needed

⅓ cup melted dark chocolate (70% cacao or higher)

½ teaspoon ground cinnamon or Chinese five-spice powder (optional)

1. Preheat the oven to 350°F.

2. Spread the pecans in an even layer on a rimmed baking sheet. Roast for about 11 minutes, or until they are deep brown in color and fragrant.

3. Remove the nuts from the oven and let cool for about 10 minutes, or until still warm but cool enough to handle. Transfer to a food processor and process until they turn to butter, stopping to scrape down the sides as needed. Depending on your processor, this will take several minutes.

4. Add 1 teaspoon of salt, the chocolate, and cinnamon (if using) and blend again. Taste and add more salt as desired.

Serving tip: A tablespoon or two of this nut butter makes a wonderful dessert by itself, or it can be used on pancakes or muffins, or mixed into a smoothie.

Per Serving (2 tablespoons): Calories: 228; Total Fat: 22g; Cholesterol: 0mg; Sodium: 110mg; Carbs: 6g; Sugar: 2g; Fiber: 4g; Protein: 3g

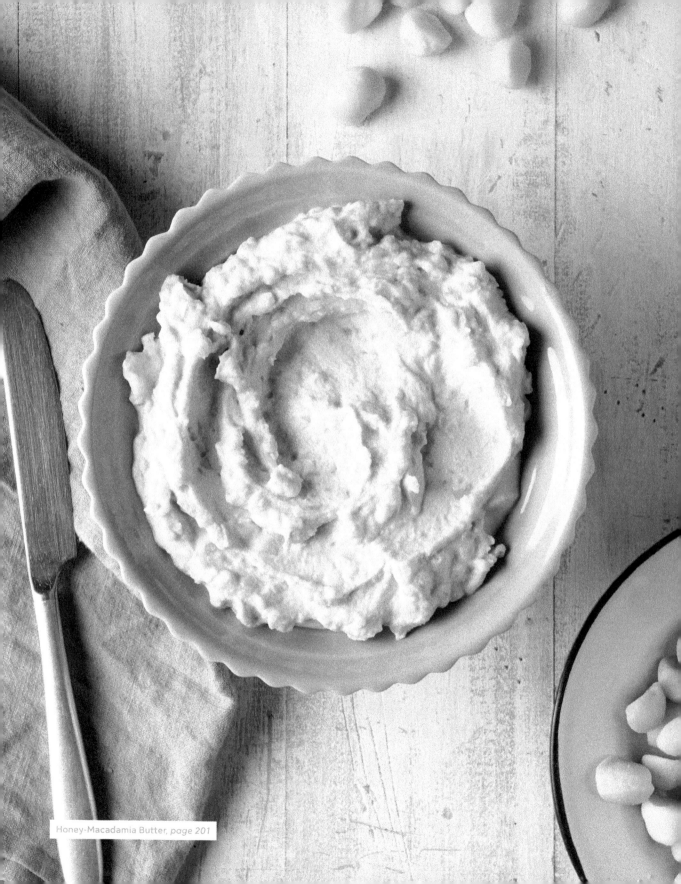

Honey-Macadamia Butter, *page 201*

15

Basic Staples, Condiments, Dressings, and More

Honey-Ginger Simple Syrup

This simple syrup can be used to make cold drinks like Ginger Limeade (page 174) or be added to hot water to create a sweet ginger tea. Clover honey has a ratio of 50/50 glucose to fructose and therefore is low FODMAP. Many people tolerate clover honey. Always buy verified honeys as many cheaper kinds are cut with high-fructose corn syrup.

Makes 1½ cups
PREP TIME: **5 minutes**
COOK TIME: **40 minutes**

1 cup water

1 cup pasteurized clover honey, raw sugar, or unrefined whole cane sugar

¼ cup coarsely chopped peeled fresh ginger

1. In a small saucepan over high heat, combine the water, honey, and ginger and cook just until boiling.

2. Reduce the heat to medium-low and simmer for 5 minutes.

3. Remove from the heat and let cool for 30 minutes.

4. Strain the syrup through a fine-mesh strainer into a glass jar; discard the ginger. Keep refrigerated.

Ingredient tip: Fresh herbs, such as basil or thyme, can be substituted for the ginger, or the simple syrup can be made with just the sweetener and water.

Per Serving (2 to 3 tablespoons, made with clover honey):
Calories: 84; Total Fat: 0g; Cholesterol: 0mg; Sodium: 2mg; Carbs: 22g; Sugar: 22g; Fiber: 0g; Protein: 0g

Chimichurri Sauce

Fresh parsley contains multiple antioxidants, so in addition to livening up your meal, this sauce is also very nutritious.

Makes 1 cup

PREP TIME: **10 minutes**

1¼ cups packed fresh parsley leaves

⅓ cup red wine vinegar

¼ cup extra-virgin olive oil

¼ cup garlic oil

¼ teaspoon sea salt

In a blender or food processor, combine the parsley, vinegar, olive oil, garlic oil, and salt. Blend until puréed. Serve immediately or let stand at room temperature until ready to serve. Keep refrigerated for up to 1 week.

Make-ahead tip: Chimichurri is an easy sauce to make, and it goes great with chicken, pork, or vegetables. To save prep time, make this sauce on the weekend and keep refrigerated for the week to add brightness to multiple dishes.

Per Serving (about 3 heaping tablespoons): Calories: 200; Total Fat: 22g; Cholesterol: 0mg; Sodium: 186mg; Carbs: 1g; Sugar: 1g; Fiber: 1g; Protein: 1g

Mustard Vinaigrette

Keep this easy vinaigrette stocked in your refrigerator. It's delicious on a variety of salads.

Makes 10 tablespoons

PREP TIME: **5 minutes**

¼ cup extra-virgin olive oil

¼ cup garlic oil

1½ tablespoons red wine vinegar

1 tablespoon freshly
squeezed lemon juice

1 rounded tablespoon Dijon or
yellow mustard (without garlic)

Salt

Freshly ground black pepper

1. In a small Mason jar, combine the olive oil, garlic oil, vinegar, lemon juice, and mustard. Cover the jar and shake well to blend.

2. Season to taste with salt and pepper. Keep refrigerated.

Preparation tip: Once you get used to making your own vinaigrette, you'll wonder why you ever liked store-bought versions. Taste your vinaigrette and add a bit more salt, vinegar, or oil to your liking.

Per Serving (2 tablespoons): Calories: 193; Total Fat: 22g; Cholesterol: 0mg; Sodium: 60mg; Carbs: 0g; Sugar: 0g; Fiber: 0g; Protein: 0g

Caesar Salad Dressing

This dressing is delicious when used on a salad (like Chicken Caesar Salad, page 102), as a dip for raw or lightly steamed vegetables, or mixed into a chopped chicken salad with julienned carrots and chopped bell peppers.

Makes about 2 cups

PREP TIME: **10 minutes**

2 large eggs (see Tip below)

2 large egg yolks (see Tip below)

2 tablespoons freshly squeezed lemon juice

1 teaspoon wild-caught anchovy paste

½ teaspoon freshly ground black pepper

¼ teaspoon sea salt

2 tablespoons organic grass-fed butter, melted

1 cup avocado oil

2 tablespoons garlic oil

¼ cup freshly grated Parmesan cheese (optional)

1 teaspoon finely chopped fresh parsley or ¼ teaspoon dried parsley

1. In a blender, combine the eggs, egg yolks, lemon juice, anchovy paste, pepper, and salt. Blend on medium speed until incorporated.

2. Add the butter and blend again.

3. With the blender running, slowly add the avocado oil and garlic oil, making sure all of the oil is incorporated. The dressing will continue to thicken. Transfer to a storage container.

4. Stir in the Parmesan cheese (if using) and parsley. Keep refrigerated for up to 1 week.

Ingredient tip: Consuming raw eggs may increase your risk of foodborne illness. You can substitute pasteurized eggs, if desired.

Per Serving (2 tablespoons): Calories: 175; Total Fat: 19g; Cholesterol: 52mg; Sodium: 688mg; Carbs: 0g; Sugar: 0g; Fiber: 0g; Protein: 2g

Ranch Dressing

If you can wait, this dressing is even better once it sits overnight. It's great on lettuce or chicken salads and makes a delicious vegetable dip.

Makes about 1 cup

PREP TIME: **10 minutes**

1 cup 24-Hour Yogurt (page 84)

¼ cup finely grated Parmesan cheese

2 tablespoons garlic oil

1 tablespoon dried chives or 3 tablespoons chopped fresh chives

1 teaspoon dried parsley or 1 tablespoon chopped fresh parsley

½ teaspoon sea salt, plus more as needed

Freshly ground black pepper

In a Mason jar or small bowl, combine the yogurt, Parmesan cheese, garlic oil, chives, parsley, and salt. Season to taste with pepper. Stir to combine the ingredients. Taste the dressing and add more salt or pepper as needed. Keep refrigerated for up to 1 week.

Ingredient tip: The salt is part of what transforms this from tasting like plain yogurt to a ranch dressing, so it's best not to leave it out; add more as desired.

Per Serving (1 tablespoon): Calories: 28; Total Fat: 3g; Cholesterol: 1mg; Sodium: 62mg; Carbs: 0g; Sugar: 0g; Fiber: 0g; Protein: 1g

Romesco Sauce

Bell peppers are on the Environmental Working Group's "Dirty Dozen" list—indicating the fruits and vegetables that are best purchased as organic because they tend to be conventionally grown with a lot of pesticides (see also the Low-FODMAP Dirty Dozen, page 204). Try romesco sauce on roasted vegetables or chicken.

Makes about 1¼ cups

PREP TIME: **10 minutes**

1 (8-ounce) jar roasted organic red bell peppers (without garlic)

⅓ cup slivered almonds, toasted

2 tablespoons organic tomato paste

2 tablespoons red wine vinegar or rice vinegar

2 tablespoons chopped fresh parsley

1 teaspoon smoked paprika (optional)

3 tablespoons garlic oil

3 tablespoons extra-virgin olive oil

Salt

Freshly ground black pepper

1. In a food processor or blender, combine the roasted peppers, almonds, tomato paste, vinegar, parsley, and paprika (if using). Purée until a thick paste forms.

2. With the machine running, add the garlic oil and olive oil and process until smooth.

3. Season to taste with salt and pepper. If the texture is too thick, add a little water to thin the sauce as needed. Use immediately or keep refrigerated for up to 1 week. Romesco sauce can also be frozen for later use.

Preparation tip: You can roast your own fresh bell peppers at home if you have time. There are numerous videos online that show various simple methods.

Per Serving (¼ cup): Calories: 216; Total Fat: 21g; Cholesterol: 0mg; Sodium: 248mg; Carbs: 6g; Sugar: 1g; Fiber: 4g; Protein: 2g

Zesty Arugula Pesto

Pesto is a wonderfully versatile condiment. Use it on zucchini noodles, roasted vegetables, rice pasta, or chicken, or serve with crackers.

Makes about 1 cup

PREP TIME: **10 minutes**

¼ cup garlic oil

⅓ cup extra-virgin olive oil

1 (6-ounce) bag organic arugula

¼ cup chopped pine nuts
  or walnuts (optional)

¼ cup grated Parmesan
  cheese (optional)

1 tablespoon freshly
  squeezed lemon juice

Salt

In a blender or food processor, combine the garlic oil, olive oil, arugula, the pine nuts and Parmesan cheese (if using), and the lemon juice. Process until the pesto is smooth, scraping down the sides as needed. Season to taste with salt. Keep refrigerated for up to 1 week.

Ingredient tip: If you don't tolerate cheese or nuts, omit them from this recipe.

Per Serving (¼ cup, made with pine nuts and cheese): Calories: 389; Total Fat: 40g; Cholesterol: 6mg; Sodium: 144mg; Carbs: 5g; Sugar: 1g; Fiber: 2g; Protein: 7g

Honey-Macadamia Butter

Soaking nuts can reduce antinutrients such as phytic acid, tannins, lectins, and oxalates. Reducing these antinutrients makes the nuts more easily digestible so that their nutrients are better absorbed. Making this macadamia butter does take some time, but it's fairly easy.

Makes 2 cups
PREP TIME: **2 hours**
COOK TIME: **12 hours**

2 cups raw macadamia nuts

1 teaspoon sea salt, divided
(½ teaspoon optional when
processing the butter)

4 cups cold water

2 tablespoons pasteurized clover
honey or maple syrup (optional)

½ teaspoon ground
cinnamon (optional)

2 tablespoons coconut oil or
avocado oil, melted (optional)

1. In a medium bowl, combine the macadamia nuts and ½ teaspoon of salt. Cover with the cold water and stir once to distribute the salt. Let the nuts soak for 2 hours.

2. Drain, rinse, and dry the nuts.

3. Transfer the nuts to a rimmed baking sheet or dehydrator tray and preheat the oven or set a dehydrator to 150°F.

4. Cook the nuts in the oven or dehydrator for 12 hours.

5. Transfer the cooked nuts to a food processor and add the honey and cinnamon (if using), and the remaining ½ teaspoon of salt if desired. Process for about 5 minutes, or until the nuts turn into butter. If the mixture is too thick, add the melted coconut oil to reach your desired consistency.

Preparation tip: If the macadamia butter is going to be consumed over a couple of days, you can omit Steps 3 and 4. Keep the nut butter refrigerated.

Per Serving (2 tablespoons, made with clover honey and coconut oil):
Calories: 123; Total Fat: 13g; Cholesterol: 0mg; Sodium: 56mg; Carbs: 4g; Sugar: 4g; Fiber: 0g; Protein: 2g

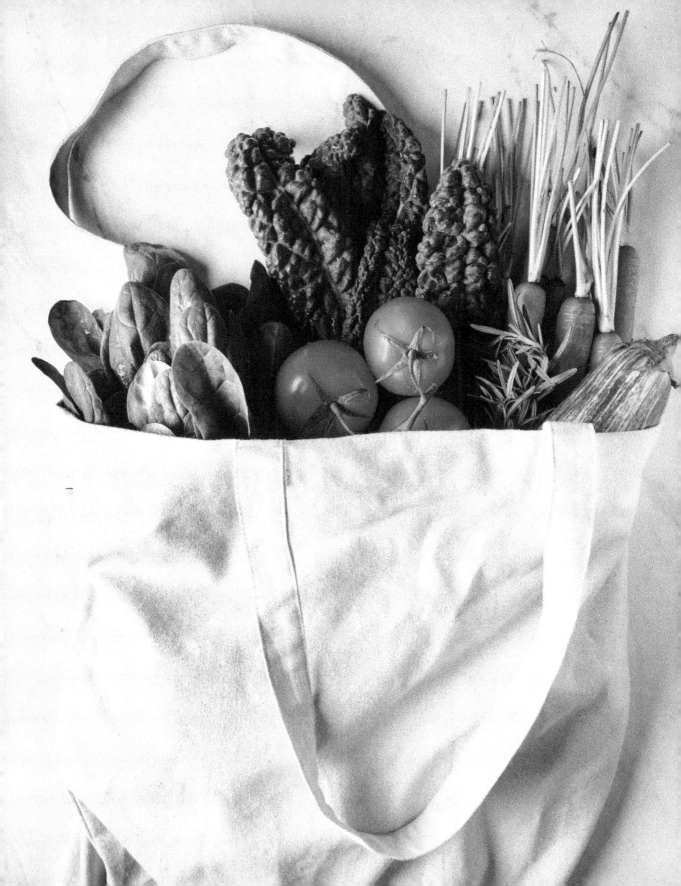

Measurement and Conversion Tables

Standard	US Standard (ounces)	Metric (approximate)
2 tablespoons	1 fl. oz.	30 mL
¼ cup	2 fl. oz.	60 mL
½ cup	4 fl. oz.	120 mL
1 cup	8 fl. oz.	240 mL
1½ cups	12 fl. oz.	355 mL
2 cups or 1 pint	16 fl. oz.	475 mL
4 cups or 1 quart	32 fl. oz.	1 L
1 gallon	128 fl. oz.	4 L

Fahrenheit (F)	Celsius (C) (approximate)
250°	120°
300°	150°
325°	165°
350°	180°
375°	190°
400°	200°
425°	220°
450°	230°

Standard	Metric (approximate)
⅛ teaspoon	0.5 mL
¼ teaspoon	1 mL
½ teaspoon	2 mL
¾ teaspoon	4 mL
1 teaspoon	5 mL
1 tablespoon	15 mL
¼ cup	59 mL
⅓ cup	79 mL
½ cup	118 mL
⅔ cup	156 mL
¾ cup	177 mL
1 cup	235 mL
2 cups or 1 pint	475 mL
3 cups	700 mL
4 cups or 1 quart	1 L

Standard	Metric (approximate)
½ ounce	15 g
1 ounce	30 g
2 ounces	60 g
4 ounces	115 g
8 ounces	225 g
12 ounces	340 g
16 ounces or 1 pound	455 g

THE LOW-FODMAP DIRTY DOZEN™

These lists are adapted from the Environmental Working Group's (ewg.org) Dirty Dozen and Clean 15 lists, tailored to include only low-FODMAP fruits and vegetables. NOTE: Some of these are high FODMAP in specific amounts so be sure to check.

The Dirty Dozen are the fruits and vegetables best purchased as organic because, if conventionally grown, they contain a lot of pesticides. This list is in order of most to least contaminated:

1. Strawberries

2. Spinach

3. Grapes

4. Celery

5. Tomatoes

6. Sweet bell peppers

7. Potatoes

8. Cucumbers

9. Cherry tomatoes

10. Lettuce

11. Blueberries, domestic

12. Kale and collard greens

THE LOW-FODMAP CLEAN 7 (NORMALLY CLEAN 15)

This list has been reduced to seven low-FODMAP fruits and vegetables that are relatively low in pesticides. These are safe to buy as conventionally grown and are listed starting with the least contaminated in the group. NOTE: Some of these are high FODMAP in specific amounts so be sure to check.

1. Avocado

2. Pineapple

3. Cabbage

4. Eggplant

5. Honeydew melon

6. Kiwi

7. Cantaloupe

Resources

WEBSITES

Bristol Stool Scale: https://www.webmd.com/digestive-disorders
/poop-chart-bristol-stool-scale
A general scale for evaluating bowel movements.

Environmental Working Group: www.ewg.org
Source for the annual Dirty Dozen and Clean 15 lists, their guide to the fruits and vegetables with the most and least amount of pesticides.

- **Dirty Dozen:** www.ewg.org/foodnews/dirty_dozen_list.php#.Wl0V8FQ-dTY

- **Clean 15:** www.ewg.org/foodnews/clean_fifteen_list.php#.WmoN2TFy5Yc

Monash University Low-FODMAP Diet app: www.monashfodmap.com/i-have-ibs
/get-the-app/
This app offers the most up-to-date and scientifically tested FODMAP list available.

SIBO—Small Intestine Bacterial Overgrowth: www.SIBOinfo.com
Dr. Allison Siebecker's website is a wealth of free information about SIBO.

The World's Healthiest Foods: www.whfoods.com/index.php
The George Mateljan Foundation is a not-for-profit foundation whose mission is to help you eat and cook for optimal health.

Vital Food Therapeutics: www.vitalfoodtherapeutics.com
Kristy Regan's site offers free SIBO-friendly recipes and information.

FOODS

Casa de Santé Low FODMAP Vegetable Stock Powder: http://bit.ly/2m84oPx

Collagen hydrolysate: Great Lakes Collagen Hydrolysate or Vital Proteins Collagen Peptides, both available on Amazon.

FODY, Low FODMAP Food Co.: www.fodyfoods.com/collections/all
Source for low-FODMAP prepared foods.

Garlic Oil Recommendations: https://fodmapeveryday.com/commercial-garlic
-infused-oils/

Gut Rx Gurus Low-FODMAP Bone Broth: https://gutrxbonebroth.com/

Histamine Intolerance Awareness Food List: www.histamineintolerance.org.uk/about
/the-food-diary/the-food-list/
A guide to low-histamine foods to help you manage your diet and health.

Living Network's High- and Low-Sulfur (Thiols) Foods: www.livingnetwork.co.za
/chelationnetwork/food/high-sulfur-sulphur-food-list/

Seeking Health Liquid Lactase Drops: www.seekinghealth.com/advancedsearch
/result/?q=lactase+drops
Provides support for lactose and dairy digestion.

WORKSHOPS, RETREATS, AND CONFERENCES

Integrative SIBO Conference: www.synergycmegroup.com/2018-integrative-sibo
-conference

Russell Delman: www.russelldelman.com
Workshops and retreats for developing presence and gratitude.

SIBO SOS Summits: http://sibosos.pages.ontraport.net/home

SIBO Symposium at National University of Natural Medicine (NUNM):
http://career-alumni.nunm.edu/continuing-education/

TESTING

QuinTron SIBO Testing: www.breathtests.com
Call to ask about testing in your area, including in-person breath tests. A list of labs in the
United States can also be found at www.siboinfo.com/testing.html.

References

Chedid, V., S. Dhalla, J.O. Clarke, et al. "Herbal Therapy Is Equivalent to Rifaximin for the Treatment of Small Intestinal Bacterial Overgrowth." *Global Advances in Health and Medicine* 3, no. 3 (May 2014): 16–24. doi:10.7453/gahmj.2014.019.

Cho E., J.M. Seddon, B. Rosner, W.C. Willett, S.E. Hankinson. "Prospective Study of Intake of Fruits, Vegetables, Vitamins, and Carotenoids and Risk of Age-Related Maculopathy." *Archives of Ophthalmology* 122, no. 6 (June 2004): 883–92. doi:10.1001/archopht.122.6.883.

Dukowicz, Andrew C., Brian E. Lacy, and Gary M. Levine. "Small Intestinal Bacterial Overgrowth." *Gastroenterology & Hepatology* 3, no. 2 (February 2007): 112–122.

Foster, Jane A., and Karen-Anne McVey Neufeld. "Gut-Brain Axis: How the Microbiome Influences Anxiety and Depression." *Trends in Neurosciences* 36, no. 5 (May 2013): 305–12. doi:10.1016/j.tins.2013.01.005.

Gareau, M.G., E. Wine, D.M. Rodrigues, et al. "Bacterial Infection Causes Stress-Induced Memory Dysfunction in Mice. *Gut* 60, no. 3 (March 2011): 307–17. doi:10.1136/gut.2009.202515.

Kasper, Kerrie L., Jean Soon Park, Charles R. Brown, et. al. "Pigmented Potato Consumption Alters Oxidative Stress and Inflammatory Damage in Men." *Journal of Nutrition* 141 no. 1 (January 1, 2011): 108–111. doi:10.3945/jn.110.128074.

Kelesidis, Theodoros, and Charalabos Pothoulakis. "Efficacy and Safety of the Probiotic *Saccharomyces Boulardii* for the Prevention and Therapy of Gastrointestinal Disorders." *Therapeutic Advances in Gastroenterology* 5, no. 2 (March 2012): 111–125. doi:10.1177/1756283X11428502.

Neufeld, K.M., N. Kang, J. Bienenstock, and J.A. Foster. "Reduced Anxiety-Like Behavior and Central Neurochemical Change In Germ-Free Mice." *Neurogastroenterology & Motility* 23, no. 3 (March 2011): 255–64. doi:10.1111/j.1365-2982.2010.01620.x.

Ojetti, V. et. al. "The Effect of Lactobacillus Reuteri Supplementation in Adults with Chronic Functional Constipation: A Randomized, Double-Blind, Placebo-Controlled Trial." *Journal of Gastrointestinal and Liver Diseases* 23, no. 4 (December 2014): 387–91. doi:10.15403/jgld.2014.1121.234.elr.

Patel, B., R. Schutte, P. Sporns, et. al. "Potato Glycoalkaloids Adversely Affect Intestinal Permeability and Aggravate Inflammatory Bowel Disease." *Inflammatory Bowel Diseases* 8, no. 5 (September 2002): 340-6.

Pimentel, M., E.J. Chow, and H.C. Lin. "Eradication of Small Intestinal Bacterial Overgrowth Reduces Symptoms of Irritable Bowel Syndrome." *The American Journal of Gastro-enterology* 95, no. 12 (December 2000): 3503–6. doi:10.1111/j.1572-0241.2000.03368.x.

Pimentel, M., E.J. Chow, and H.C. Lin. "Normalization of Lactulose Breath Testing Correlates with Symptom Improvement in Irritable Bowel Syndrome. A Double-Blind, Randomized, Placebo-Controlled Study." *The American Journal of Gastroenterology* 98, no. 2 (February 2003): 412–9. doi:10.1111/j.1572-0241.2003.07234.x.

Rezaie, Ali, Michelle Buresi, et. al. "Hydrogen and Methane-Based Breath Testing in Gastrointestinal Disorders: The North American Consensus." *The American Journal of Gastroenterology* 112 (May 2017): 775-784. https://www.ncbi.nlm.nih.gov/pubmed/28323273.

Riso, Patrizia, Francesco Visioli, Simona Grande, et. al. "Effect of a Tomato-Based Drink on Markers of Inflammation, Immunomodulation, and Oxidative Stress." *Journal of Agricultural and Food Chemistry* 54, no. 7 (April 2006): 2563–2566. doi:10.1021/jf053033c/.

Wilson, Dédé. "Know What's in Your Garlic Oil." FODMAP Everyday. Accessed December 14, 2017. www.fodmapeveryday.com/know-whats-garlic-oil/.

Xiao, Z., G.E. Lester, Y. Luo, Q. Wang. "Assessment of Vitamin and Carotenoid Concentrations of Emerging Food Products: Edible Microgreens." *Journal of Agricultural and Food Chemistry* 60, no. 31 (August 2012): 7644-7651. doi:10.1021/jf300459b.

Zoran I., B.Y. Avital, P. Yaccov, et. al. "Total Antioxidant Activity (TAA) of Bell Pepper During Prolonged Storage on Low Temperature." *Journal of Agricultural Sciences* 53, no.1 (January 2008). doi:10.2298/JAS0801003I.

Meal Index

Recipe Index

Index

Acknowledgments

First and foremost, this book is for all those suffering from digestive disorders throughout the world. Healing is possible.

Thank you to my clients, from whom I learn every day. You bring humor, joy, and light to my work, and there's nowhere else I'd rather be.

I am deeply grateful for mentorship from Dr. Allison Siebecker and Dr. Steven Sandberg-Lewis. Their kindness and wisdom are immeasureable, and they have been extremely instrumental in my learning and growth as a practitioner. I am privileged to be part of a dedicated community of SIBO-focused doctors, nutritionists, and health practitioners.

Many thanks to Shivan Sarna for your insight, grit, and deep caring. Blessings and thanks to Russell Delman for teaching me the wisdom of presence. Thank you to Karen Davis for your nutritional analysis acumen and friendship. My appreciation to Areej Khataebeh for seeing parts of me that are just coming into focus.

My appreciation to everyone at Callisto Media.

Many thanks to my loving, supportive, and crazy friends.

Much love and gratitude to my husband for keeping me sane during this process. To my parents, siblings, stepchildren, nieces, nephews, aunts, uncles, and cousins, thank you for being there. We are a family of teachers and writers, and I am honored to be part of it. To my nephew Joel, thank you for believing in the nutrition empire—maybe you'll get the dedication in the next book if you text me more.

And, lastly, thank you to my mom for inspiring my love of cooking and lifelong learning.

About the Author

KRISTY REGAN, of Vital Food Therapeutics, specializes in working with clients who have digestive disorders, including SIBO, IBS, IBD, and leaky gut. Her practice combines nutritional therapy, lifestyle education, and counseling to assist clients in their healing journeys.

Kristy was diagnosed with SIBO when little information was available. This led to a multiyear journey in SIBO research, developing her own inner authority, discovering new ways to cook, and creating delicious new recipes.

She appreciates how important it is to address both physical and emotional health. She is also aware of the role gratitude and presence play in supporting us in feeling whole while we are in the midst of healing.

She is passionate about sharing her insights and expertise in cooking, nutrition, health, and mind-body therapies via podcasts, classes, and speaking engagements. Kristy is available for individual nutrition and wellness appointments via Skype worldwide. Visit her website, VitalFoodTherapeutics.com for free recipes and digestive health information.